Sarcoidosis and Granulomatosis - Diagnosis and Management

Edited by Mohammad Hosein K. Motamedi

Published in London, United Kingdom

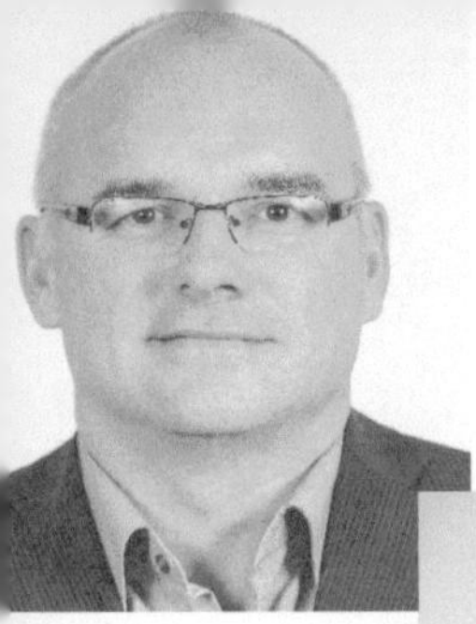
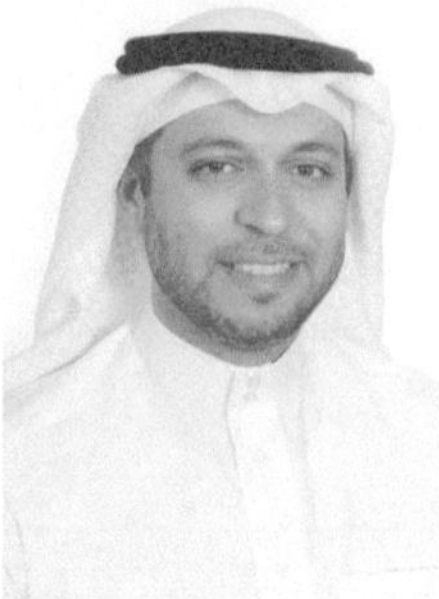
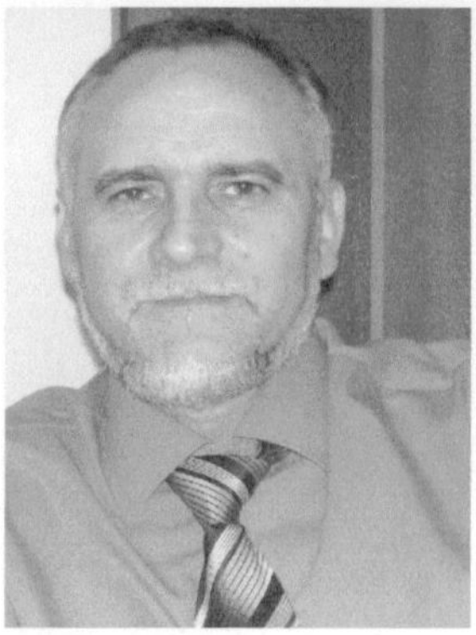
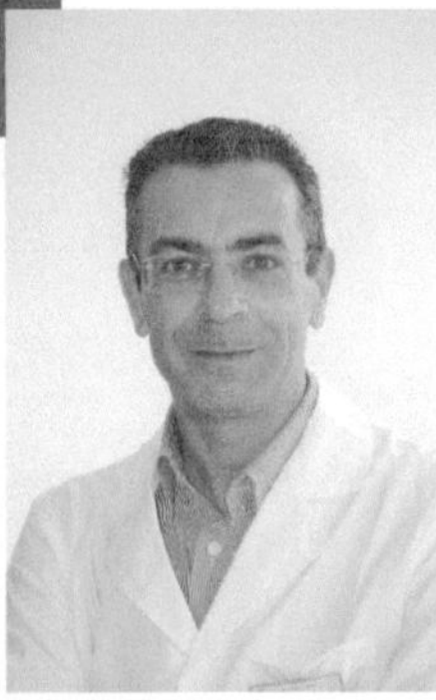
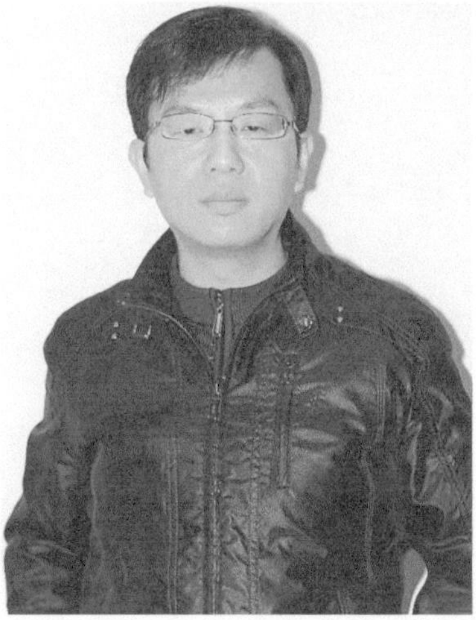
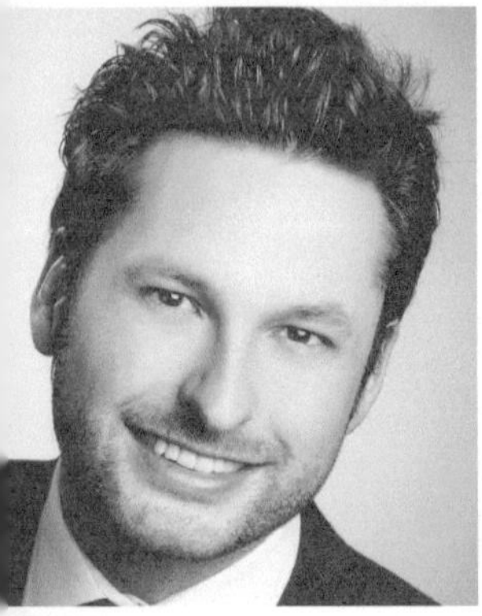
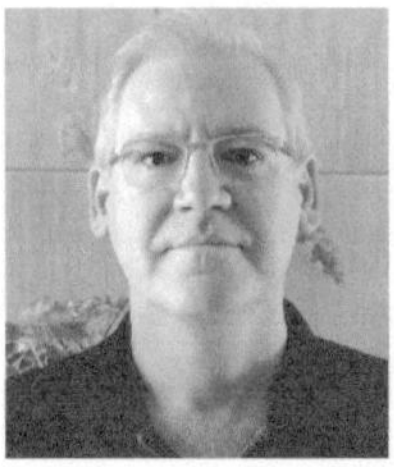

IntechOpen

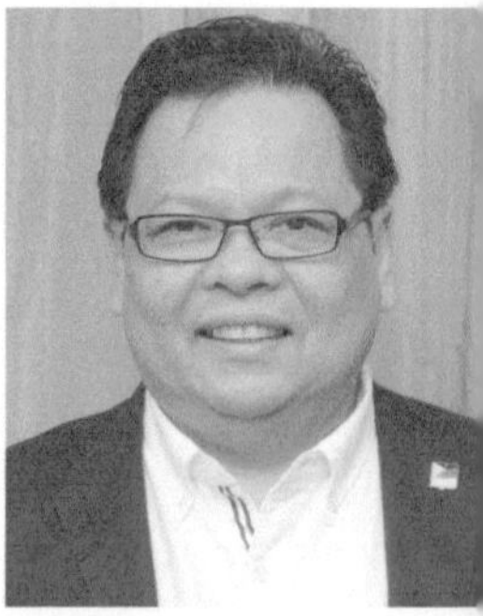
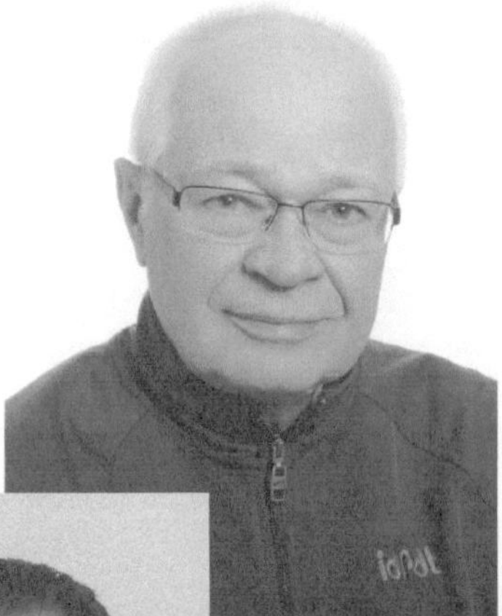
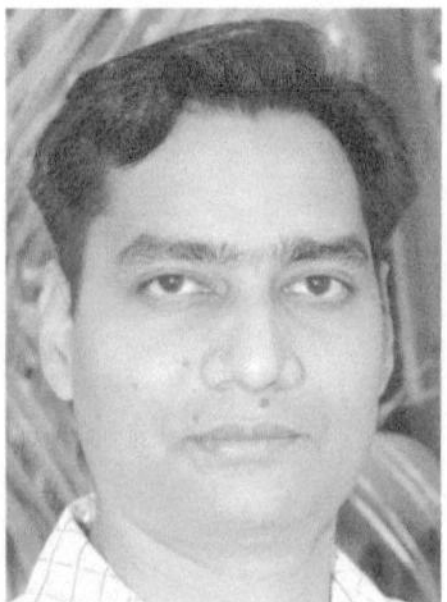
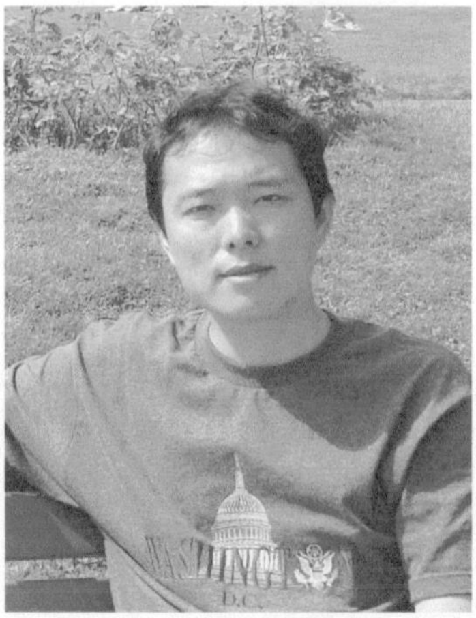
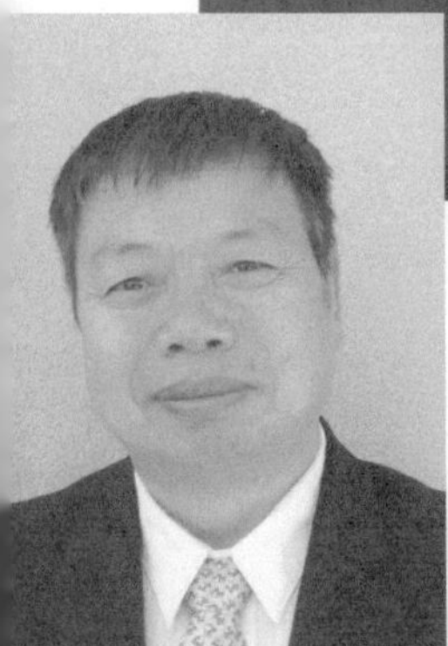
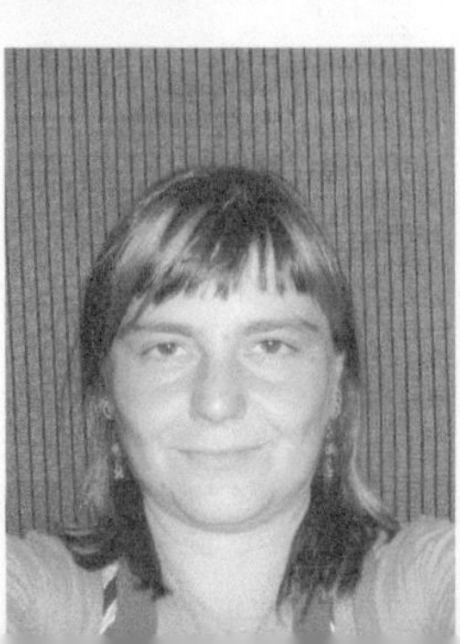

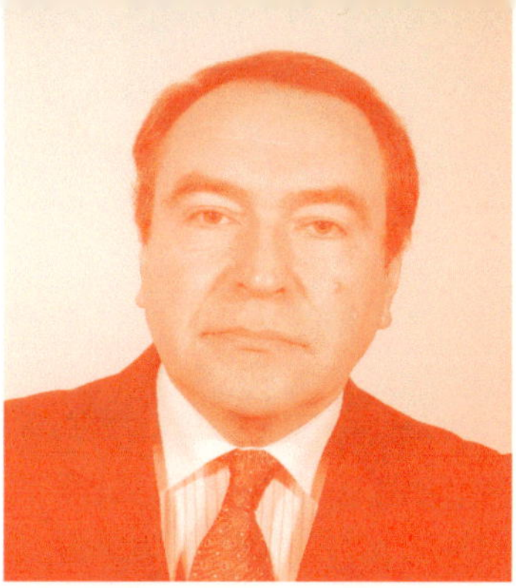
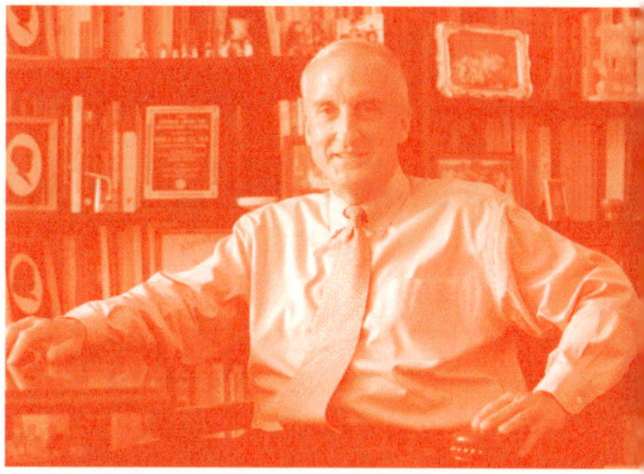
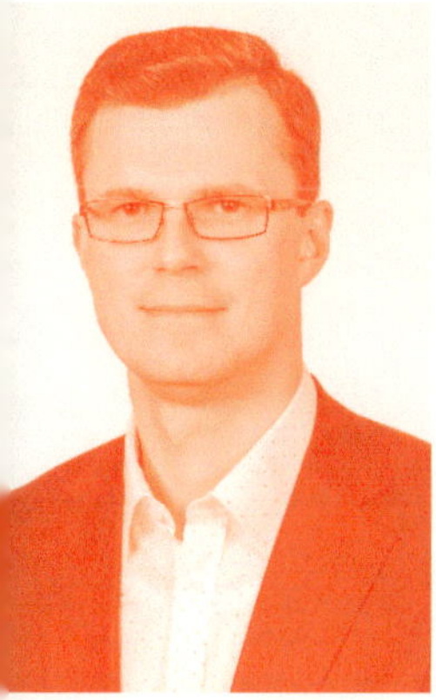
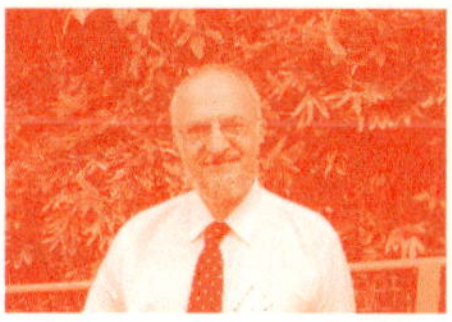
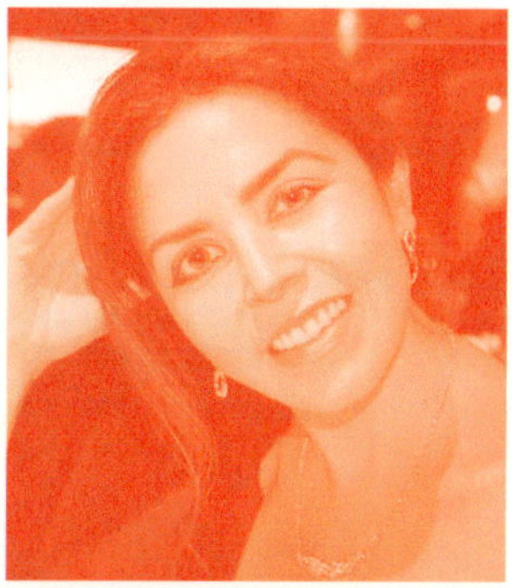

Supporting open minds since 2005

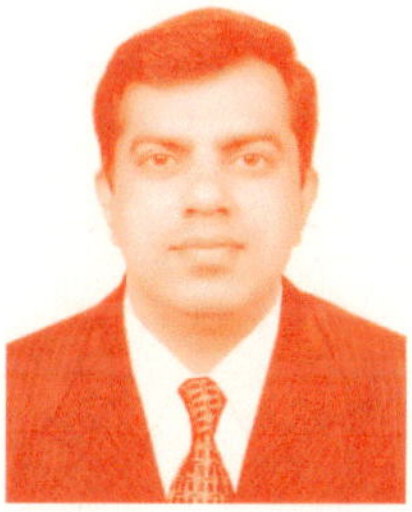
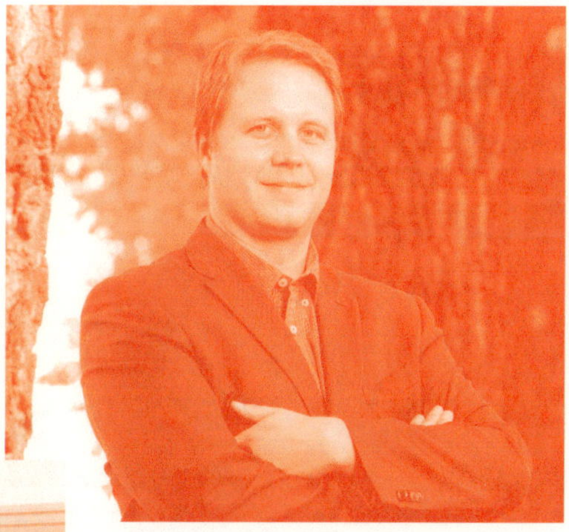
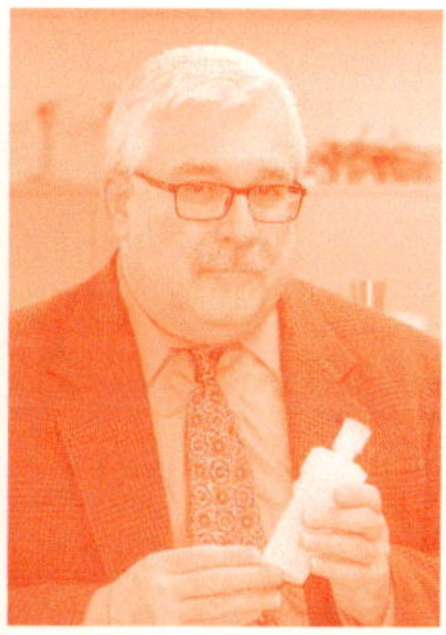
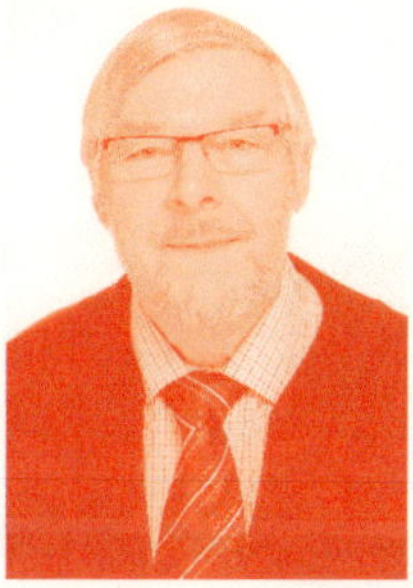
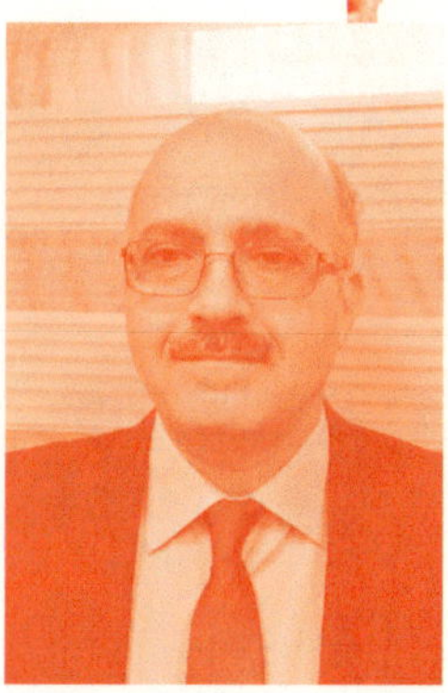
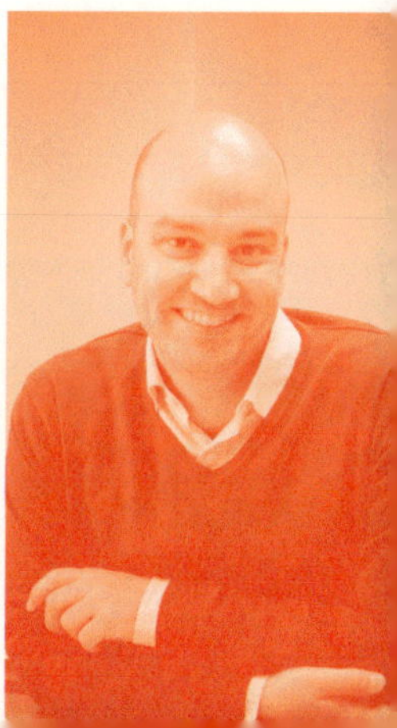
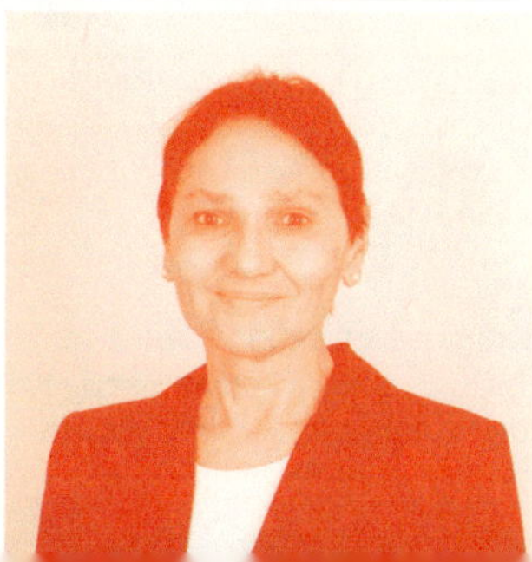

Sarcoidosis and Granulomatosis - Diagnosis and Management
http://dx.doi.org/10.5772/intechopen.73968
Edited by Mohammad Hosein K. Motamedi

Contributors
Galina Makovetskaya, Lilia Mazur, Elena Balashova, Angel Robles-Marhuenda, Jhan Carlos Altamar, Miguel Tejeda, Mohammad Hosein Kalantar Motamedi, Ahmed Fahim, Rajarajan Anandavelu, Maccarone Marica Tina, Patricia Lopez Arribas, Elena Martinez Gomez, Álvaro Zapico Goñi, Maria Viktorovna Samsonova, Laura Iliescu, Letitia Toma, Jae Y. Ro, Komal Arora, Neeraj Kaur, Suchibrata Das, Sharareh Kamfar, Taghi Azizi, Andrey L. Chernyaev

First published in London, United Kingdom, 2020 by IntechOpen
IntechOpen is the global imprint of INTECHOPEN LIMITED, registered in England and Wales, registration number: 11086078, 7th floor, 10 Lower Thames Street, London, EC3R 6AF, United Kingdom
Printed in Croatia

British Library Cataloguing-in-Publication Data
A catalogue record for this book is available from the British Library

Additional hard and PDF copies can be obtained from orders@intechopen.com

Sarcoidosis and Granulomatosis - Diagnosis and Management
Edited by Mohammad Hosein K. Motamedi
p. cm.
Print ISBN 978-1-83881-035-1
Online ISBN 978-1-83962-833-7
eBook (PDF) ISBN 978-1-83962-834-4

For EU product safety concerns:
IN TECH d.o.o., Prolaz Marije Krucifikse Kozulić 3, 51000 Rijeka, Croatia, info@intechopen.com or visit our website at intechopen.com.

Meet the editor

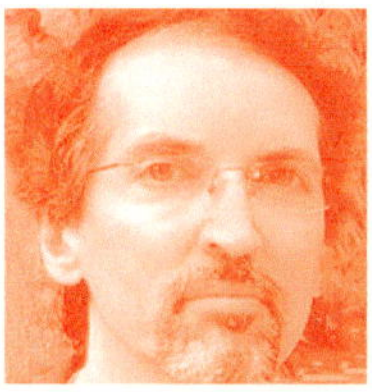

Dr. Mohammad Hosein Kalantar Motamedi is a Professor of Oral and Maxillofacial Surgery at the Trauma Research Center, BMSU, and attending faculty of OMF Surgery at the Azad University of Medical Sciences, Tehran. He received his American Diploma from Pennington High School, in Pennington, VA, USA (honor student) and his Iranian Diploma from Hurr High School in Tehran (honor student). After graduation he was accepted at the University of Houston, Texas, USA where he studied predent. Two years later he transferred to the University of Tehran College of dentistry where he received his Doctorate of Dental Surgery Degree (DDS). He completed his Residency in Oral and Maxillofacial Surgery at SBUMS from 1987-1991, and was valedictorian of the National Board Exams in 1991. In 1995 he completed his fellowship at the University of Basel, Switzerland; he obtained full Professorship in 2007. He has published 25 books, 61 international conferences proceedings, supervised 63 doctorate dissertations, and published 185 papers indexed in PUBMED with an h-index of 21. He is Editor-in-Chief of TRAUMA MONTHLY journal and one of the founders of the BMSU Trauma Research Center and more recently the Craniomaxillofacial Research Center. He was granted 1st place prize at the Bagher Alum National Research Festival in 2010 and awarded 2nd Place Prize at the 16th International Razi Research Festival on Medical Sciences. The Iranian Society of OMF Surgeons awarded him "Most Published" in 2009 and 2010, and he was chosen for membership in the National Elite Foundation. In 2013 he was accepted in the Academy of Medical Sciences and he is listed in the Marquis Book 'Who's Who in the World" (1999-2020).

Contents

Preface

Sarcoidosis is a multi-organ, granulomatous disease the etiology of which remains unknown; it is characterized by T-cell dysfunction and B-cell hyperactivity with increased local immune activity and inflammation that leads to the formation of noncaseating granulomas in the organs involved. The lung and lymphatic system are the most commonly affected organs, however, virtually any organ may be affected. Other common sites of involvement include the skin, eye, central nervous system, and the heart. Patients may present different symptoms related to the disease stage and the specific organ involved.

Sarcoidosis is a global disease, and its prevalence has increased twofold over the past years. Due to the clinical heterogeneity and variable diagnostic criteria in different countries, it is difficult to calculate the exact prevalence and incidence of sarcoidosis. Age, sex, race, and geographic origin significantly influence the incidence of sarcoidosis. The book at hand is an international text on sarcoidosis. It is the fruition of specialists from several countries. The chapters presented herein are written by experts in this field. The book is organized in a logical manner starting with an introductory chapter, followed by diagnostic techniques, imaging, differential diagnosis, clinical manifestations, and then involvement of specific organs, followed by granulomatous diseases mimicking sarcoidosis.

I would like to take the opportunity to thank all my national and international colleagues who helped me compile the chapters necessary for this book. I sincerely hope that it will be of use to all clinicians involved in the treatment of this mysterious disease.

Mohammad Hosein K. Motamedi, DDS
Professor of Oral and Maxillofacial Surgery,
BMSU, IAUMS, TUMS Trauma and Craniomaxillofacial Research Centers,
Tehran, Iran

Chapter 1

Introductory Chapter: Orofacial Sarcoidosis and Noncaseating Granulomatosis

Shareh Kamfar, Taghi Azizi and Mohammad Hosein Kalantar Motamedi

1. Introduction

Sarcoidosis is a multi-organ, granulomatous disease of unknown etiology characterized by T-cell dysfunction and B-cell hyperactivity with increased local immune activity and inflammation that leads to the formation of noncaseating granulomas in the organs involved [1]. The lung and lymphatic system are the most commonly affected organs, but virtually any organ may be affected [2]. Other common sites of involvement include the skin, eye, central nervous system (CNS), and the heart [3]. Patients may present with different symptoms related to the disease stage and the specific organ involved [4]. Sarcoidosis is a global disease, and its prevalence has increased twofold over the past years [5]. Due to the clinical heterogeneity and variable diagnostic criteria in different countries, it is difficult to calculate the exact prevalence and incidence of sarcoidosis. Age, sex, race, and geographic origin significantly influence the incidence rate of sarcoidosis [6]. A definite diagnosis of the disease when an identifiable etiology and definitive diagnostic criteria is lacking remains challenging [3].

2. Types

2.1 Head and neck sarcoidosis

This may occur in combination with, or independent of, CNS sarcoidosis; this has been found in 10–15% of patients with systemic disease [7].

2.2 Orofacial sarcoidosis

Although orofacial presentations of sarcoidosis are uncommon, it is important because of the fact that sarcoidosis in the orofacial region may indicate the development of systemic involvement [4]. Generally, in the case of orofacial sarcoidosis, swelling of the salivary glands is observed. Xerostomia may or may not be present; and bilateral enlargement of the parotid glands may be affected in 4–6% of the cases [8].

2.3 Orofacial granulomatosis

Orofacial granulomatosis (OFG), defined by Wiesenfeld in 1985, encompasses conditions characterized by non-necrotizing granulomatous inflammation of soft tissues in the oral and maxillofacial region that present clinically with labial enlargement, perioral and/or mucosal swelling, oral ulcerations, gingivitis, and a variety of other orofacial features [9]. The clinical manifestations can be highly variable, and this variability makes it difficult to diagnose. OFG is a disease that encompasses a broad range of presentations, which may include oral manifestations of a systemic condition such as Crohn's disease (CD), sarcoidosis, granulomatosis with polyangiitis, and Melkersson-Rosenthal syndrome [10]. On the other hand, some studies say that OFG displays a spectrum of diseases ranging from granulomatous cheilitis to patients with granulomas involving other orofacial tissues, with or without facial nerve palsy and plicated tongue (Melkersson-Rosenthal syndrome) [11]. According to recent evidence, OFG can also be classified into three categories [12, 13], namely:

- OFG alone
- OFG with intestinal CD
- OFG with gastrointestinal granulomata but no symptoms of intestinal CD.

3. Etiology

The exact cause of OFG is yet to be elucidated, although various etiological agents have been proposed such as genetic predisposition, contact allergies, various microbiological agents, and immunologic causes [9]. The role of genetic predisposition has been evaluated in different studies, but there is a lack of conclusive evidence between HLA and pathogenesis of orofacial granulomatosis [14–16]; there is no evidence to support genetics causes for OFG [16]. Because of involvement of OFG in CD and sarcoidosis, the possible role of infections in the pathogenesis of OFG has been suggested [17]. Several studies have suggested that there is no conclusive evidence to support the role for allergy in OFG [18]. Recently, a monoclonal lymphocytic expansion in OFG lesion has been identified that may be responsible for the granuloma formation through cytokine production in lesions [19, 20].

4. Presentation

The diagnosis of OFG is based on clinical presentation, but it can be highly variable. The clinical features of OFG are mainly similar to orofacial manifestations of CD without apparent lesions in the bowels and may also mimic orofacial manifestations of sarcoidosis [21] labial enlargement, and sometimes oral ulcers are the main clinical features of OFG [22].

4.1 Lips

The lips are the most common sites of involvement in OFG. Labial swelling can involve the lower or upper lip or both. This feature of OFG is persistent but may eventually become recurrent. Each episode in this inflammatory process usually lasts several weeks to months [23]. The swelling varies in consistency from soft to rubbery [24].

4.2 Oral lesions

Three types of oral ulcers may occur in OFG as follows [25]:

- Chronic and deep ulcers in the buccal or labial vestibules with surrounding raised borders (most common).

- Superficial aphthous-like ulcers on any oral mucosal surface (less common).

- Pustules on the anterior gingivae and/or labial vestibules or soft palate (the least common).

4.3 Salivary gland

In asymptomatic patients, enlargement of the salivary glands is the first identifiable sign of the disease [8]. Involvement of salivary glands has been reported in the maxillofacial region that xerostomia or bilateral parotid swelling is the result of this involvement [26, 27]. Inflammation of salivary glands differentiates OFG from other granulomatous diseases such as cheilitis glandularis, Wegener's granulomatosis, sarcoidosis, and deep fungal infections [28].

5. Diagnosis

Since sarcoidosis is a multi-organ disorder, it can be difficult to diagnose with a single specific diagnostic test; and also, the presence of noncaseating granulomas alone does not confirm the presence of the disease because many other diseases can cause granulomas. On the other hand, these structures can be formed in various disorders [29]. In as much as in most cases of sarcoidosis, oral involvement often appears as the first manifestation of the disease; in diagnosis, the following criteria are considered [30]:

- Symptomatic oral manifestations

- Clinical and radiological findings compatible with a diagnosis of systemic sarcoidosis

- Pathologic evidence of noncaseating granulomas in the soft tissues of the oral cavity

- Exclusion of other causes of oral granulomatosis by histology of oral tissue biopsy negative for fungus

- No clinical evidence of other granulomatous diseases.

5.1 Differential diagnosis

As mentioned above, because of the same clinical features of orofacial lesions in granulomatous diseases, differential diagnoses must be considered for such diseases and other conditions including [31]:

- **Infections**, including tuberculosis, syphilis, leprosy, cat-scratch disease, and mycosis.

- **Crohn's disease** with the development of ulcers in the GI tract as the main manifestation.

- **Wegener's disease**, an uncommon necrotizing granulomatosis condition with a set of clinical manifestations with a different immunopathogenesis [32].

- **Foreign body granulomas**, formation of noncaseating granulomas and also labial and mucosal swellings with foreign bodies as the main characteristics of the disease [28].

- **OFG**, a condition that is restricted to the orofacial region (some diseases such as Crohn's disease, sarcoidosis, cheilitis granulomatosa, Wegener's granulomatosis, granulomatous infections, etc. can mimic its features), specifically lip swelling [33].

5.2 Diagnostic tests

Due to the ambiguity and difficulty in the exact diagnosis of granulomatous diseases and OFG, appropriate clinical and laboratory tests as well as radiographic and endoscopic investigations and also staining techniques and biopsy can be helpful to differentiate between such diseases.

Useful evaluations for differentiating granulomatous diseases include, as follows [28]:

- Biopsy: useful for the correct diagnosis.

- Microscopic investigations: for detection of granulomatous inflammation.

- Special stains: used to rule out deep fungal infections and bacterial infections.

- Polarized light microscopy: for identification of foreign bodies in the tissues.

- Chest radiography and assessment of serum levels of angiotensin-converting enzyme (ACE); complete blood count, erythrocyte sedimentation rate (ESR), and serum levels of folic acid, iron, and vitamin B12; and tuberculin skin test are done to assess whether a systemic disease is responsible for the granulomatous inflammation or not.

- Gastrointestinal evaluation is essential, especially in the presence of signs of anemia and intestinal malabsorption.

OFG: Blood tests, hemoglobin, C-1 esterase inhibitor, serum iron and transferrin, chest X-ray, and GI endoscopy/histopathology should be normal, and tuberculin skin test, PAS reaction and Ziehl-Neelsen stain, and polarized light microscopy for identification of foreign body materials should be negative. Also, noncaseating inflammation as well as elevated IgG and serum angiotensin-converting enzyme (ACE) levels are seen in this disease.

Crohn's disease: There are GI symptoms, decreased vitamin B12 and ferritin and increased CRP. Blood test, abdominal radiography, endoscopy, and colonoscopy should be considered.

Sarcoidosis: There are clinical symptoms, anemia, and also increased ESR, CPR, serum ACE, serum, and urinary calcium in sarcoidosis patients. Chest radiograph as well as negative microbial culture and negative staining are also helpful in diagnosis.

Wegener's granulomatosis: Clinical symptoms, vasculitis, and necrotizing granulomatosis are seen in this disease. Chest and sinus radiography as well as kidney function test anti-neutrophil cytoplasmic antibody (ANCA) and ESR should be done.

Tuberculosis: Caseating granuloma is seen in the disease. Ziehl-Neelsen staining, chest X-ray, PPD, and PAS test are used for diagnosis.

Leprosy: Granulomatous inflammation is present in this disease, and for more accurate diagnosis, PAS and acid-fast staining are done.

Foreign body granulomas: Noncaseating granulomatosis and foreign bodies are evident in this disease.

Cheilitis granulomatosa (CG): There is no evidence of GI involvement. Blood tests, chest radiography, and acid-fast staining should be done. Serum calcium and ACE and ESR are checked.

5.3 Histopathology

Histopathologic evaluation is one of the useful methods in OFG diagnosis. Several studies have demonstrated that OFG and Crohn's disease are similar with regard to their orofacial features and histopathology or may be similar to other granulomatous diseases; so it can be said that OFG is a diagnosis of exclusion [22]. Therefore, other complementary techniques like special stains for fungal infections or Ziehl-Neelsen for bacterial infections, negative microbial culture for sarcoidosis, etc. should be done to exclude other causes of granulomatous conditions.

Histopathological evidences indicate that in OFG lesions, noncaseating granulomas may not be present in all cases (from 43 to 82%) [11, 34–37] (**Figures 1** and **2**). Dilated lymphatics, edema of corium, slight fibrosis, with/without multiple noncaseating granulomas with Langerhans giant cells, and lymphocytes may be seen in OFG lesions [11] (**Figures 3** and **4**).

5.4 Treatment of OFG

The definite treatment of the disease in the lack of a causative factor remains to be elucidated. The first line in treatment is the use of local or systemic corticosteroids or both. Corticosteroids are effective in reducing facial swelling and preventing recurrence. Patients with mild swelling are treated locally [35]. Atrophy and hypopigmentation are the only side effects of local treatment, but side effects in the use of corticosteroids systemically are more important and must be avoided because of chronicity and recurrence of the disease and long-term nature of complications [38]. The use of triamcinolone 10 mg/ml is also often suggested in the treatment of local swellings of the lips [39].

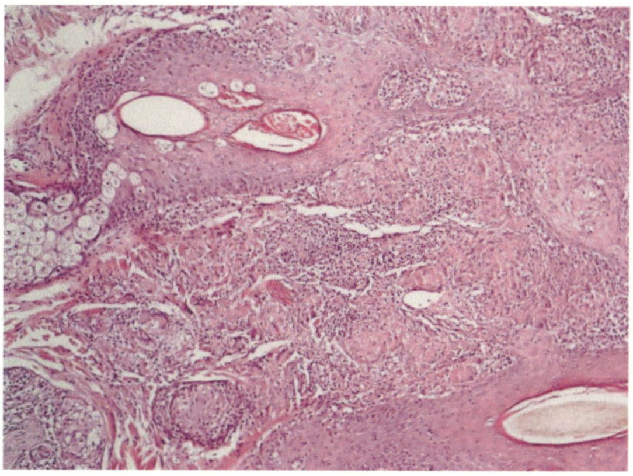

Figure 1.
Noncaseating granulomas of sarcoidosis in skin (H&E low power).

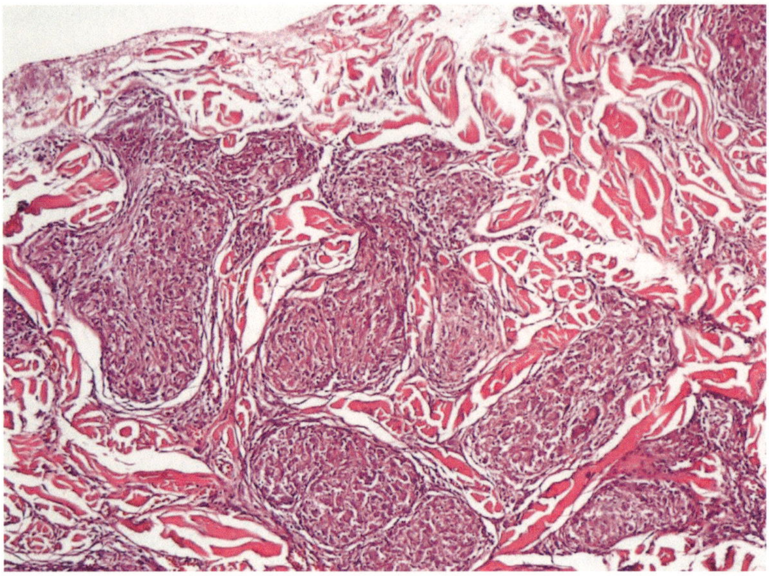

Figure 2.
Confluent noncaseating granulomatosis of sarcoidosis.

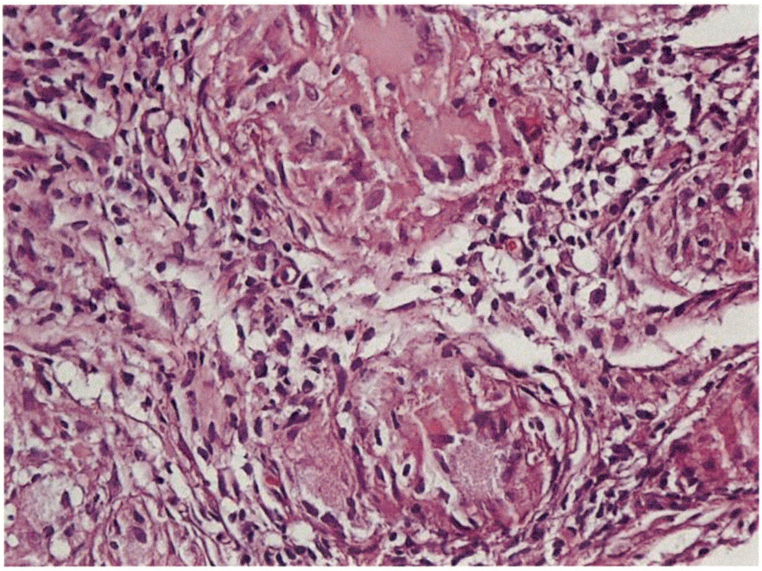

Figure 3.
Asteroid bodies and multinucleated giant cells in sarcoidosis.

Other suggested treatments for OFG in the literature include hydroxychloroquine [35, 40], methotrexate, clofazimine [35], metronidazole, minocycline [41] alone or in combination with oral prednisone, thalidomide [42, 43], dapsone, and danazol. Surgery may be used in cases that do not respond to medical treatment. Altogether, a good prognosis is predicted for OFG.

5.5 Prognosis

The pattern of onset in orofacial sarcoidosis in patients determines the course and prognosis of the disease and also therapeutic effects after treatment [44],

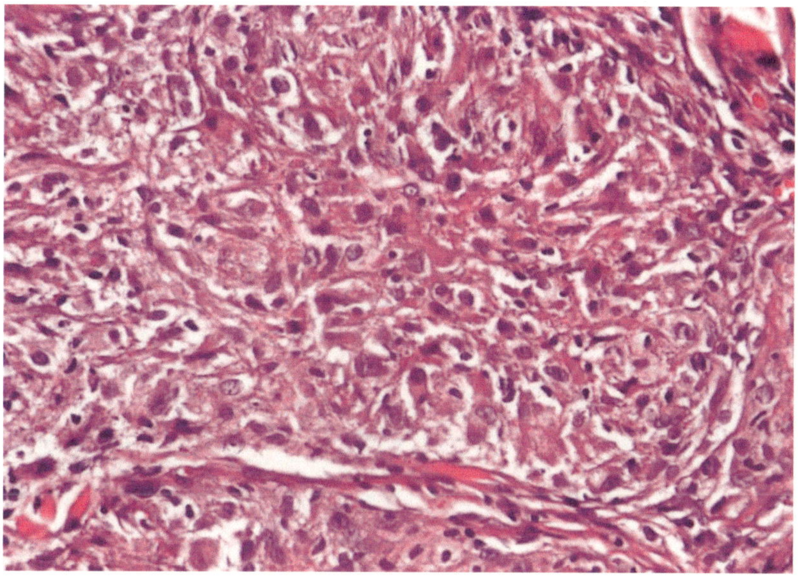

Figure 4.
Asteroid bodies and multinucleated giant cells in sarcoidosis (High-power view).

although affected patients may have a variety of nonspecific symptoms or may be asymptomatic. Oral involvement has been considered as the initial feature of the disease [45]. Although orofacial features in this disease are rare, a wide range of presentations indicates development of systemic involvement in present or future, so it must be considered. This disorder usually appears in the second and third decades of life [46] with no known racial predilection. In addition, it should be taken into consideration that women are more susceptible than men in this disease [47]. Moreover, death from sarcoidosis is a rare phenomenon except in special circumstances such as terminal fibrosis in the lungs, heart, or CNS [48]. Many patients with sarcoidosis (two-thirds) generally have a remission within a decade after diagnosis, with or without consequences.

6. Discussion

OFG is a rare disorder with unknown etiology. As mentioned, there are a variety of causative agents for OFG; but according to the accumulating data, there is no conclusive scientific evidence for the role of genetic susceptibility to the disease in the literature; so in this context, further studies are necessary [49]. Because of histopathological and clinical overlap in oral lesions of granulomatous diseases such as Crohn's disease, sarcoidosis, CG, foreign body granulomas, tuberculosis, etc. [50, 51], there is a controversial question between clinicians and pathologists that whether the formation of granulomas in the oral lesions is a distinct disease or just a feature of a systemic disease. OFG patients should be monitored for all of the symptoms in order to strengthen the possibility of OFG by exclusion of additional symptoms [28].

6.1 Organ involvement

Sarcoidosis is a multisystem disorder that may affect any organ system such as the lungs, lymph nodes, skin, eyes, liver, heart, and nervous, musculoskeletal, renal, and endocrine systems [52]. The lungs are the site of involvement and granuloma formation [52]; 90% of patients have clinical manifestation of sarcoidosis in the lungs [53]. Oral involvement has been considered as the first feature of the disease although intraoral presentations of sarcoidosis and also tongue sarcoidosis are particularly rare and uncommon [54]. Sarcoidosis signs and symptoms vary depending on which organs are affected and also the stage of the disease [4].

6.2 Disease course

Disease course of sarcoidosis is usually favorable. Patients with asymptomatic organ involvement have a high rate of spontaneous resolution that often happens within 6 months of onset [3, 55]. Every 3 months in the first year after diagnosis, follow-up visits need to be carried out and after that once a year for 3–5 years in patients without problems [3, 56, 57]. In patients having a disease course that is progressive, immunosuppressive treatment is recommended. Long-term corticosteroids in patients must be limited because of major problems such as obesity and development of complicated metabolic syndrome [56, 58]. Mortality in sarcoidosis is low [59].

6.3 Diagnosis of exclusion

Without definitive diagnostic criteria, diagnosis of sarcoidosis requires exclusion of other granulomatous diseases such as tuberculosis, Crohn's disease, etc. [3]; therefore systemic disease evidence as well as compatible clinical and radiological abnormality, histological confirmation of noncaseating granulomas, and exclusion of other granulomatous diseases (that are able to present similar histological and clinical features) can be useful in the diagnosis [60].

6.4 Laboratory markers

Serum angiotensin-converting enzyme (ACE) is the first widely used marker that has been used as diagnostic and prognostic marker of sarcoidosis but has low specificity as a marker because of its poor predictive value [61–63]. In sarcoidosis, ACE is released by pulmonary endothelial cells into blood vessels to perform its functions. ACE is elevated in affected patients [64]. Serum ACE levels are currently considered as a marker of granuloma formation with limited sensitivity and specificity, and because of its limitation, it must be investigated with other markers in sarcoidosis. As mentioned before, ACE can be used for diagnosis and follow-up, but it must be correlated with clinical phenotypes and radiological findings [65]. In addition, several markers of inflammation that can be involved in the pathogenesis of the sarcoidosis have also been reported, which include lysozyme, cytokines, chemokines, and various molecules produced by activated macrophages or lymphocytes [66–68].

6.5 Pattern of onset

Sarcoidosis have been known as a time-limited disease with disease course of 1–3 years in half of the patients, less than 5 years in most remaining cases, and rarely for decades [69].

Abrupt onset is the characteristics of acute sarcoidosis, while chronic sarcoidosis has a progressive onset. According to the annual organ screening tests, most types of organ involvement in sarcoidosis occur within 2 years of the onset of disease [70]. For treatment and prognosis of sarcoidosis, mode of onset is one of the most valid factors [71].

6.6 Treatment outcome

Appropriate decision for treatment in sarcoidosis is difficult especially in the absence of a causative agent. Sarcoidosis treatment is proposed on the basis of prevalence of asymptomatic organ involvement, rate of spontaneous resolution, and complications of long-term corticosteroids therapy [3, 56]. There is a general rule that if only organ function is threatened, organ involvement should be treated [56, 57, 69]. Laboratory testing, biopsy, imaging studies, physical examination, and any other diagnostic tests are required before any treatment. For example, pulmonary function tests and stress testing are required before any treatment for pulmonary sarcoidosis [56]. Corticosteroid therapy is considered the first line in treatment for acute and chronic sarcoidosis and may be used alone or with other medications [57, 72]. Treatment of sarcoidosis is variable between asymptomatic cases and severe cases with systemic corticosteroid therapy [4]. For patients with neurological or ocular involvement or progressive respiratory disease, systemic therapy is prescribed [4]. Immunosuppressive combination therapy is the second line in treatment of sarcoidosis in order to limit the corticosteroid dose [55]. Accumulating evidence suggests that systemic corticosteroids should be used for at least 6 months and then should be reduced gradually [57].

7. Conclusion

OFG is an uncommon immunologically mediated disorder with unknown etiology that affects the soft tissues of the oral and maxillofacial region. Although the precise cause of OFG is still unknown, allergy, infection, and genetic predisposition as well as immunological reaction have been suggested as probable causes that can be effective in pathogenesis of OFG. Clinical features of OFG are nonspecific, and various presentations in disease make it difficult to diagnose, so a comprehensive clinical, laboratory, and microscopic evaluation is required for exact diagnosis and treatment [28]. A number of granulomatous disorders, such as deep fungal infections, tuberculosis, angioedema, leprosy, Wegener's granuloma, Crohn's disease, and sarcoidosis, are similar to OFG in clinical features specifically persistent lip swelling, so differential tests are needed for diagnosis of OFG [33]. Because of similarity between OFG and some of the granulomatous diseases, this point arises that whether or not OFG is a distinct clinical disorder [12]. In this context, further studies are needed to differentiate OFG from this group of disorders.

Author details

Sharareh Kamfar[1], Taghi Azizi[2] and Mohammad Hosein Kalantar Motamedi[3,4*]

1 Hamedan University of Medical Sciences, Hamedan, Iran

2 Baqiyatallah University of Medical Sciences, Tehran, Iran

3 Baqiyatallah University of Medical Sciences, Trauma Research Center, Tehran, Iran

4 Islamic Azad University of Medical Sciences, College of Dentistry, Craniomaxillofacial Research Center, Tehran, Iran

*Address all correspondence to: motamedical@yahoo.com

References

[1] Patterson KC, Strek ME. Pulmonary fibrosis in sarcoidosis. Clinical features and outcomes. Annals of the American Thoracic Society. 2013;**10**(4):362-370

[2] Iannuzzi MC, Fontana JR. Sarcoidosis: Clinical presentation, immunopathogenesis, and therapeutics. Journal of the American Medical Association. 2011;**305**(4):391-399

[3] Baughman RP, Culver DA, Judson MA. A concise review of pulmonary sarcoidosis. American Journal of Respiratory and Critical Care Medicine. 2011;**183**(5):573-581

[4] Poate T, Sharma R, Moutasim KA, Escudier M, Warnakulasuriya S. Orofacial presentations of sarcoidosis—A case series and review of the literature. British Dental Journal. 2008;**205**(8):437

[5] Erdal BS, Clymer BD, Yildiz VO, Julian MW, Crouser ED. Unexpectedly high prevalence of sarcoidosis in a representative US metropolitan population. Respiratory Medicine. 2012;**106**(6):893-899

[6] Nunes H, Soler P, Valeyre D. Pulmonary sarcoidosis. Allergy. 2005;**60**(5):565-582

[7] Dash GI, Kimmelman CP. Head and neck manifestations of sarcoidosis. The Laryngoscope. 1988;**98**(1):50-53

[8] Mandel L, Kaynar A. Sialadenopathy: A clinical herald of sarcoidosis: Report of two cases. Journal of Oral and Maxillofacial Surgery. 1994;**52**(11):1208-1210

[9] Rana AP. Orofacial granulomatosis: A case report with review of literature. Journal of Indian Society of Periodontology. 2012;**16**(3):469

[10] Mignogna MD, Fedele S, Lo Russo L, Lo Muzio L. Orofacial granulomatosis with gingival onset. Journal of Clinical Periodontology. 2001;**28**(7):692-696

[11] Al Johani KA, Moles DR, Hodgson TA, Porter SR, Fedele S. Orofacial granulomatosis: Clinical features and long-term outcome of therapy. Journal of the American Academy of Dermatology. 2010;**62**(4):611-620

[12] Sanderson J, Nunes C, Escudier M, Barnard K, Shirlaw P, Odell E, et al. Oro-facial granulomatosis: Crohn's disease or a new inflammatory bowel disease? Inflammatory Bowel Diseases. 2005;**11**(9):840-846

[13] White A, Nunes C, Escudier M, Lomer MC, Barnard K, Shirlaw P, et al. Improvement in orofacial granulomatosis on a cinnamon-and benzoate-free diet. Inflammatory Bowel Diseases. 2006;**12**(6):508-514

[14] Satsangi J, Jewell D, Rosenberg W, Bell J. Genetics of inflammatory bowel disease. Gut. 1994;**35**(5):696

[15] Gibson J, Wray D. Human leucocyte antigen typing in orofacial granulomatosis. British Journal of Dermatology. 2000;**143**(5):1119-1121

[16] Meisel-Stosiek M, Hornstein O, Stosiek N. Family study on Melkersson-Rosenthal syndrome. Some hereditary aspects of the disease and review of literature. Acta Dermato-Venereologica. 1990;**70**(3):221-226

[17] O'Neill R, Penman R. 'Sarcoidosis' complicated with nocardiosis. Journal of the Irish Medical Association. 1969;**62**(386):287

[18] Troiano G, Dioguardi M, Giannatempo G, Laino L, Testa NF, Cocchi R, et al. Orofacial granulomatosis: Clinical signs of different pathologies. Medical Principles and Practice. 2015;**24**(2):117-122

[19] Lim S, Stephens P, Cao Q, Coleman S, Thomas D. Molecular analysis of T cell receptor beta variability in a patient with orofacial granulomatosis. Gut. 1997;**40**(5):683-686

[20] De JQ, Cordel N, Bravard P, Lenormand B, Joly P, editors. Miescher's cheilitis and lymphocytic clonal expansion: 2 cases. Annales de Dermatologie et de Vénéréologie; Jan 2004. **131**(1 Pt 1):7-55

[21] Wiesenfeld D, Ferguson M, Mitchell D, MacDonald D, Scully C, Cochran K, et al. Oro-facial granulomatosis—A clinical and pathological analysis. QJM: An International Journal of Medicine. 1985;**54**(1):101-113

[22] Leao J, Hodgson T, Scully C, Porter S. Orofacial granulomatosis. Alimentary Pharmacology & Therapeutics. 2004;**20**(10):1019-1027

[23] Odukoya O. Orofacial granulomatosis: Report of two Nigerian cases. The Journal of Tropical Medicine and Hygiene. 1994;**97**(6):362-366

[24] Mignogna MD, Fedele S, Lo Russo L, Lo Muzio L. The multiform and variable patterns of onset of orofacial granulomatosis. Journal of Oral Pathology & Medicine. 2003;**32**(4):200-205

[25] Clayden AM, Bleys CM, Jones SF, Saage NW, Aldred MJ. Orofacial granulomatosis: A diagnostic problem for the unwary and a management dilemma. Case reports. Australian Dental Journal. 1997;**42**(4):228-232

[26] Clayman L, MacLennan M, Dolan RL. Nonpainful swelling of the palate and loosening of the maxillary incisors. Journal of Oral and Maxillofacial Surgery. 1998;**56**(11):1327-1335

[27] Abul A, Onadeko B, Khadadah M, Behbehani N, Cerna M, Cherian J, et al. Clinical patterns of diffuse parenchymal lung disease in Kuwait: A prospective study. Medical Principles and Practice. 2004;**13**(2):78-83

[28] Javadzadeh A, Pakfetrat A, Falaki F, Seyyedi S. Approach to orofacial granulomatosis and review of literature. Journal of Islamic Dental Association of IRAN (JIDAI). 2012;**24**(3):3

[29] Costabel U, Guzman J, Drent M. Diagnostic approach to sarcoidosis. European Respiratory Monograph. 2005;**32**:259

[30] Bouaziz A, Le Scanff J, Chapelon-Abric C, Varron L, Khenifer S, Gleizal A, et al. Oral involvement in sarcoidosis: Report of 12 cases. QJM: An International Journal of Medicine. 2012;**105**(8):755-767

[31] Islam NM, Bhattacharyya I, Cohen DM. Common oral manifestations of systemic disease. Otolaryngologic Clinics of North America. 2011;**44**(1):161-182

[32] Swain S, Ray R. Wegener's granulomatosis of nose: A case report. Indian Journal of Otolaryngology and Head & Neck Surgery. 2011;**63**(4):402-404

[33] Neville BW, Damm DD, Chi AC, Allen CM. Oral and Maxillofacial Pathology. Oral Manifestations of Systemic Diseases. Elsevier Health Sciences; 2015:566-570

[34] Greene RM, Rogers RS III. Melkersson-Rosenthal syndrome: A review of 36 patients. Journal of the American Academy of Dermatology. 1989;**21**(6):1263-1270

[35] Van Der Waal RI, Schulten EA, Van Der Meij EH, Van De Scheur MR, Starink TM, Van Der Waal I. Cheilitis granulomatosa: Overview of 13 patients with long-term follow-up—Results of management. International Journal of Dermatology. 2002;**41**(4):225-229

[36] Kanerva M, Moilanen K, Virolainen S, Vaheri A, Pitkäranta A. Melkersson-Rosenthal syndrome. Otolaryngology–Head and Neck Surgery. 2008;**138**(2):246-251

[37] McCartan B, Healy C, McCreary C, Flint S, Rogers S, Toner M. Characteristics of patients with orofacial granulomatosis. Oral Diseases. 2011;**17**(7):696-704

[38] Mignogna M, Fedele S, Russo LL, Adamo D, Satriano R. Effectiveness of small-volume, intralesional, delayed-release triamcinolone injections in orofacial granulomatosis: A pilot study. Journal of the American Academy of Dermatology. 2004;**51**(2):265-268

[39] Sakuntabhai A, MacLeod RI, Lawrence CM. Intralesional steroid injection after nerve block anesthesia in the treatment of orofacial granulomatosis. Archives of Dermatology. 1993;**129**(4):477-480

[40] Allen CM, Camisa C, Hamzeh S, Stephens L. Cheilitis granulomatosa: Report of six cases and review of the literature. Journal of the American Academy of Dermatology. 1990;**23**(3):444-450

[41] Olivier V, Lacour J, Castanet J, Perrin C, Ortonne J. Chéilite granulomateuse chez une enfant. Archives de Pédiatrie. 2000;**7**(3):274-277

[42] Medeiros M, Araujo MI, Guimarães NS, Freitas LAR, Silva TMC, Carvalho EM. Therapeutic response to thalidomide in Melkersson-Rosenthal syndrome: A case report. Annals of Allergy, Asthma & Immunology. 2002;**88**(4):421-424

[43] Hegarty A, Hodgson T, Porter S. Thalidomide for the treatment of recalcitrant oral Crohn's disease and orofacial granulomatosis. Oral Surgery, Oral Medicine, Oral Pathology, Oral Radiology, and Endodontology. 2003;**95**(5):576-585

[44] James DG. Sarcoidosis 2001. Postgraduate Medical Journal. 2001;**77**(905):177-180

[45] Jackowski J, Dragisic D, Arnold G, Dirschka T. Primary oral sarcoidosis preceding Lofgren's syndrome. Oral Surgery, Oral Medicine, Oral Pathology, Oral Radiology, and Endodontics. 2005;**100**(2):183-185

[46] Lourenço SV, Lobo AZ, Boggio P, Fezzi F, Sebastiao A, Nico MMS. Gingival manifestations of orofacial granulomatosis. Archives of Dermatology. 2008;**144**(12):1627-1630

[47] Marcoval J, Viñas M, Bordas X, Jucglà A, Servitje O. Orofacial granulomatosis: Clinical study of 20 patients. Oral Surgery, Oral Medicine, Oral Pathology, and Oral Radiology. Apr 2012;**113**(4):e12-e17. DOI: 10.1016/j.oooo.2011.10.011

[48] Steinberg MJ, Mueller DP. Treating oral sarcoidosis. Journal of the American Dental Association (1939). 1994;**125**(1):76-79

[49] Tilakaratne W, Freysdottir J, Fortune F. Orofacial granulomatosis: Review on aetiology and pathogenesis. Journal of Oral Pathology & Medicine. 2008;**37**(4):191-195

[50] Garnuszewski Z. A case of tuberculosis of the tongue treated with streptomycin. Gruzlica (Warsaw Poland: 1926). 1949;**17**(3-4):306-308

[51] Crohn BB, Ginzburg L, Oppenheimer GD. Regional ileitis: A pathologic and clinical entity. Journal of the American Medical Association. 1932;**99**(16):1323-1329

[52] Soumithran C, Bindu R, Shahi AK, Shaikh SF. Orofacial sarcoidosis. Asian Journal of Oral and Maxillofacial Surgery. 2005;**17**(4):280-283

[53] Rotsinger J, Drake W. Sarcoidosis: Unknown etiology and genetic predisposition provides therapeutic challenges. Journal of Pulmonary and Respiratory Medicine. 2014;**4**(190):2

[54] Mendelsohn S, Field E, Woolgar J. Sarcoidosis of the tongue. Clinical and Experimental Dermatology. 1992;**17**(1):47-48

[55] Baughman RP, Judson MA. Relapses of sarcoidosis: What are they and can we predict who will get them? European Respiratory Journal. Feb 2014;**43**(2):337-339. DOI: 10.1183/09031936.00138913

[56] Valeyre D, Prasse A, Nunes H, Uzunhan Y, Brillet P, Muller-Quernheim J. Lancet. 2014;**383**:1155-1167

[57] Judson MA. The treatment of pulmonary sarcoidosis. Respiratory Medicine. 2012;**106**(10):1351-1361

[58] Grutters J, Van den Bosch J. Corticosteroid treatment in sarcoidosis. European Respiratory Journal. 2006;**28**(3):627-636

[59] Gerke AK. Morbidity and mortality in sarcoidosis. Current Opinion in Pulmonary Medicine. 2014;**20**(5):472

[60] Costabel U, Bonella F, Ohshimo S, Guzman J, editors. Diagnostic modalities in sarcoidosis: BAL, EBUS, and PET. In: Seminars in Respiratory and Critical Care Medicine. © Thieme Medical Publishers; 2010

[61] Sharma P, Smith I, Maguire G, Stewart S, Shneerson J, Brown MJ. Clinical value of ACE genotyping in diagnosis of sarcoidosis. The Lancet. 1997;**349**(9065):1602-1603

[62] Stokes G, Monaghan J, Schrader A, Glenn C, Ryan M, Morris B. Influence of angiotensin converting enzyme (ACE) genotype on interpretation of diagnostic tests for serum ACE activity. Australian and New Zealand Journal of Medicine. 1999;**29**(3):315-318

[63] Lieberman J. Elevation of serum angiotensin-converting-enzyme (ACE) level in sarcoidosis. The American Journal of Medicine. 1975;**59**(3):365-372

[64] Studdy PR, Lapworth R, Bird R. Angiotensin-converting enzyme and its clinical significance—A review. Journal of Clinical Pathology. 1983;**36**(8):938-947

[65] Schürmann M. Angiotensin-converting enzyme gene polymorphisms in patients with pulmonary sarcoidosis. American Journal of Pharmacogenomics. 2003;**3**(4):233-243

[66] Rothkrantz-Kos S, van Dieijen-Visser MP, Mulder PG, Drent M. Potential usefulness of inflammatory markers to monitor respiratory functional impairment in sarcoidosis. Clinical Chemistry. 2003;**49**(9):1510-1517

[67] Ziegenhagen M, Rothe M, Schlaak M, Müller-Quernheim J. Bronchoalveolar and serological parameters reflecting the severity of sarcoidosis. European Respiratory Journal. 2003;**21**(3):407-413

[68] Rottoli P, Bargagli E. Is bronchoalveolar lavage obsolete in the diagnosis of interstitial lung disease? Current Opinion in Pulmonary Medicine. 2003;**9**(5):418-425

[69] Hunninghake G. Statement on sarcoidosis. Joint Statement of the American Thoracic Society (ATS), the European Respiratory Society (ERS) and the World Association of Sarcoidosis and Other Granulomatous Disorders (WASOG) adopted by the ATS Board of Directors and by the ERS Executive Committee, February 1999. American Journal of Respiratory and Critical Care Medicine. 1999;**160**:736-755

[70] Prasse A. The diagnosis, differential diagnosis, and treatment of sarcoidosis. Deutsches Ärzteblatt International. 2016;**113**(33-34):565

[71] Siltzbach L, James DG, Neville E, Turiaf J, Battesti J, Sharma OP, et al. Course and prognosis of sarcoidosis around the world. The American Journal of Medicine. 1974;**57**(6):847-852

[72] Judson MA. An approach to the treatment of pulmonary sarcoidosis with corticosteroids: The six phases of treatment. Chest. 1999;**115**(4):1158-1165

Chapter 2

Current Diagnostic Techniques in Sarcoidosis

Rajarajan Anandavelu and Ahmed Fahim

Abstract

Sarcoidosis is an enigmatic disorder with a propensity for lung involvement in the majority of cases (~90%) and is characterized by noncaseating granulomatous inflammation on histological analysis. The techniques to establish the diagnosis have evolved over time, and a clear diagnostic algorithm for the clinicians dealing with this disease is desirable. Thoracic computed tomography is the imaging modality of choice in pulmonary sarcoidosis and provides accurate assessment of staging, parenchymal involvement, and response to immunomodulatory therapies. The advent of EBUS-TBNA has been a step forward with an excellent diagnostic yield in the presence of mediastinal/hilar lymphadenopathy and has replaced the traditional approach of obtaining biopsy samples via transbronchial and endobronchial routes. The preferred initial investigation for the confirmation of diagnosis is dependent on the organ involvement and the expertise available. A core biopsy of cervical lymph nodes is a less invasive and economical alternative in selected cases of suspected pulmonary sarcoidosis and warrants further evaluation in prospective manner to establish if it can be considered as a first-line investigation in all new cases suspected to have pulmonary sarcoidosis. A multidisciplinary approach is crucial for the diagnosis and management, and a simplified algorithm is proposed to help guide clinicians dealing with this disease of myriad clinical and radiological manifestations.

Keywords: sarcoidosis, granulomatous inflammation, lymphadenopathy, core biopsy, endobronchial ultrasound-guided transbronchial needle aspiration (EBUS-TBNA)

1. Introduction

Sarcoidosis is an enigmatic disorder with a propensity for lung involvement in the majority of cases (90%) and is characterized by noncaseating granulomatous inflammation on histological analysis. The techniques to establish the diagnosis have evolved over time, and a clear diagnostic algorithm for clinicians dealing with this disease is desirable. Thoracic computed tomography is the imaging modality of choice in pulmonary sarcoidosis and provides accurate assessment of the stage, parenchymal involvement, and response to immunomodulatory therapies. The advent of EBUS-TBNA has been a step forward with an excellent diagnostic yield in the presence of mediastinal/hilar lymphadenopathy and has replaced the traditional approach of obtaining biopsy samples via transbronchial and endobronchial routes. The preferred initial investigation for the confirmation of diagnosis is dependent upon the organ involved and the expertise available. A core biopsy of cervical lymph nodes is a less invasive and economical alternative in selected cases

Radiological Staging of Sarcoidosis

Stage	Chest Radiographic appearance
0	Normal
I	Lymphadenopathy only
II	Lymphadenopathy and parenchymal disease
III	Parenchymal disease only
IV	Extensive pulmonary Fibrosis

Figure 1.
Chest radiograph appearances according to stage of sarcoidosis.

of suspected pulmonary sarcoidosis and warrants further evaluation in a prospective manner to establish if it can be considered a first-line investigation in all new cases suspected to have pulmonary sarcoidosis. A multidisciplinary approach is crucial for the diagnosis and management; a simplified algorithm is proposed to help guide clinicians dealing with this disease of myriad clinical and radiological manifestations.

Sarcoidosis is a disease of uncertain etiology characterized by evidence of non-necrotizing granulomatous inflammation on histological assessment. As the disease commonly affects the lungs, the patients are likely to be referred to pulmonologists for further investigations. Chest radiography is usually the first investigation carried out in the primary care setting suggesting the possibility of hilar lymph node enlargement, and sarcoidosis has traditionally been staged according to chest radiographic appearances (**Figure 1**).

Radiological assessment of sarcoidosis has been revolutionized by high-resolution computed tomography (HRCT) scanning of lungs and is currently the best available modality to assess the extent of involvement of lung parenchyma/interstitial compartment and response to immunomodulatory therapies to evaluate alveolitis and reversibility of the disease process. The current diagnostic techniques for histological assessment in pulmonary sarcoidosis are invasive, and there is a need for a less invasive approach to obtain tissue sample(s). This chapter aims to discuss the available diagnostic techniques in sarcoidosis and propose an algorithm to the pulmonologists/radiologists and clinicians dealing with sarcoidosis as a tool to aid for reaching the diagnosis with minimally invasive investigations. It is recommended that an ultrasound-guided core biopsy of cervical lymph nodes (along with assessment of parotid glands) may be considered first-line investigation in the presence of mediastinal and or hilar lymphadenopathy, a suitable target to sample neck lymph nodes.

2. Diagnostic techniques

The diagnosis of sarcoidosis is best supported by the presence of noncaseating/necrotizing granulomatous inflammation on histological analysis, following the exclusion of other granulomatous disorders such as mycobacterial or fungal diseases on special immunohistochemical stains. The diagnostic techniques for sarcoidosis can be subclassified into four groups:

- Radiological techniques
- Bronchoscopic techniques
- Ultrasound-guided biopsy techniques
- Surgical techniques

2.1 Radiological imaging techniques

These include chest radiography, high-resolution computed tomography, and positron emission tomography (PET) scanning.

2.1.1 Chest radiography

The typical chest radiographic appearances in sarcoidosis consist of symmetric bilateral hilar and mediastinal lymphadenopathy. Fibrosis is noticed in 5–25% of patients with sarcoidosis on initial chest radiograph [1]. **Figure 2** demonstrates an example of advanced stage sarcoidosis with the development of fibrosis and parenchymal distortion.

2.1.2 High-resolution computed tomography

High-resolution computed tomography has improved the diagnostic accuracy of sarcoidosis in terms of parenchymal involvement (**Figure 3**) and assessed any reversible component such as alveolitis that may not be readily evident on chest radiography. Moreover, the abnormalities on HRCT scan do correlate better with respiratory functional impairment than chest radiograph findings [2].

Sarcoidosis is a disease with a myriad of radiological abnormalities on HRCT, including hilar and mediastinal lymphadenopathy, ground glass abnormality, and fibrosis in a peribronchovascular, perilymphatic distribution, pulmonary parenchymal nodules, and beading of the fissures. There is a mid- to upper-zone preponderance of these abnormalities and usually distributed along the bronchovascular

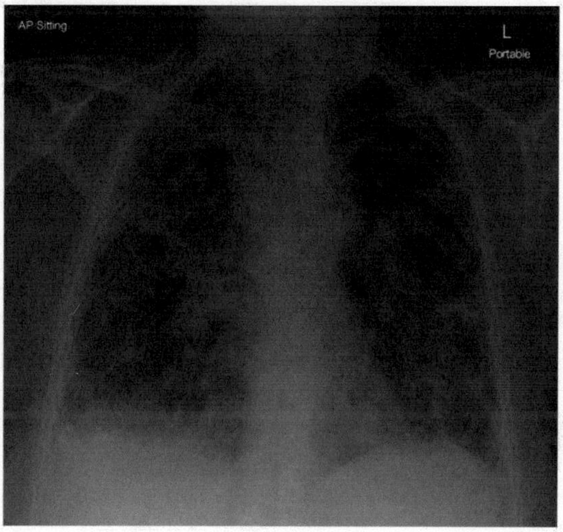

Figure 2.
Stage III sarcoidosis with evidence of hilar lymphadenopathy and parenchymal involvement.

bundles [3]. HRCT may be able to demonstrate lymphadenopathy in mediastinal distribution better than a chest radiograph and sometimes demonstrate evidence of calcification within these nodes (**Figure 4**).

The precise role of HRCT in the clinical monitoring of sarcoidosis is unknown. However, it may prove to be a useful tool to assess acute alveolitis and inflammation in selected cases of refractory sarcoidosis, where treatment decisions to commence

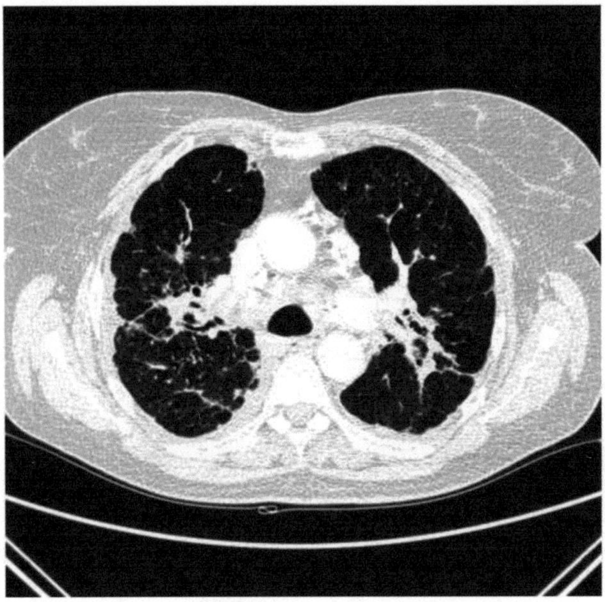

Figure 3.
Parenchymal distortion with fibrosis in a peribronchovascular distribution in bilateral upper lobes in sarcoidosis.

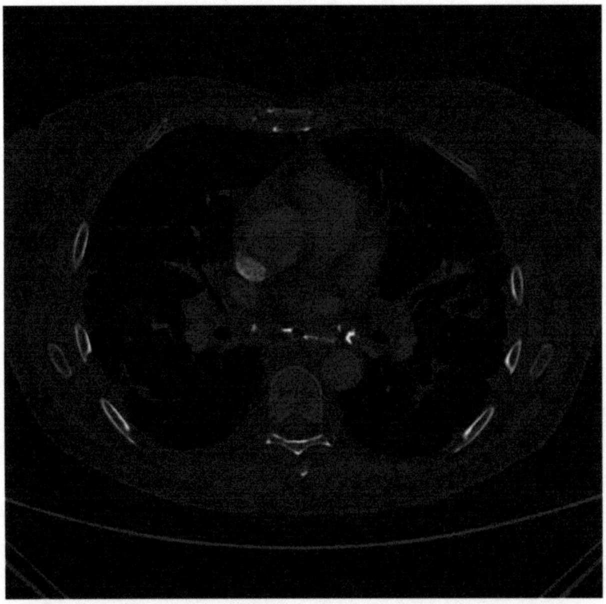

Figure 4.
Calcified mediastinal lymphadenopathy with bilateral hilar nodal enlargement in a patient with confirmed sarcoidosis.

biologic therapies such as infliximab are being made [3]. A study by De Boer et al. showed that the total extent of parenchymal disease on the CT scan on a lobar basis could predict the likelihood of transbronchial biopsy being positive following bronchoscopy [4], demonstrating its utility on diagnostic grounds.

2.1.3 Positron emission tomography scan

Positron emission tomography scan can be a useful tool to detect the extent of the disease, identify multisystem disease such as cardiac sarcoidosis, and may help to identify a desirable site for biopsy [5]. Moreover, it could be invaluable in the decision to initiate immunosuppression and assess the efficacy of treatment [6, 7]. Furthermore, it may help in predicting relapse in pulmonary sarcoidosis [8].

A retrospective study by Teirstein et al. showed that a combination of diagnostic modalities such as 18F-fluorodeoxyglucose (FDG-PET) and CT scan is more sensitive than PET-only imaging [9]. Whole-body FDG-PET was found to be significantly better in identifying occult and reversible granulomas. Moreover, a positive PET scan in isolation should not be considered as an indication for treatment. In another study by Yu et al., the sensitivity and specificity for benign and malignant disease were 94.2% and 73.8%, respectively [10]. It was, however, noted that maximum standard uptake value (SUVMax) as semiquantitative measurement alone could not be used to differentiate benign vs. malignant lesions.

The FDG-PET scan has a cumulative effect in cardiac sarcoidosis. PET scan has also been evaluated in predicting supraventricular arrhythmias, and it was noted that patients with left atrial enlargement were associated with increased likelihood of supraventricular arrhythmias [11]. Smedema et al. reported that biventricular late gadolinium enhancement was the strongest predictor of adverse outcome, and an asymptomatic myocardial scar of less than 8% in the left ventricular mass was associated with a favorable outcome in patients with pulmonary sarcoidosis [12].

On the basis of current available evidence, the role of PET-CT is limited in routine clinical care of patients with pulmonary sarcoidosis. However, it may be a useful imaging modality in multisystem sarcoidosis, in particular when the clinical suspicion for cardiac involvement is high and the diagnostic techniques such as echocardiography and or cardiac MRI have unequivocal results. Moreover, PET-CT may become a useful adjunct to assess the response to immunosuppression with corticosteroids and/or antimetabolites and may guide us to an appropriate biopsy site to sample suspected multisystem disease.

2.2 Bronchoscopic techniques

2.2.1 Bronchoalveolar lavage (BAL) and transbronchial biopsy (TBB)

Bronchoscopic techniques have been employed in the evaluation of pulmonary sarcoidosis for a very long time and have been the mainstay of histological confirmation historically. Granulomatous inflammation in sarcoidosis usually involves the bronchovascular and centrilobular structures.

Transbronchial biopsies help to obtain the histological diagnosis in support of clinical-radiological diagnosis especially when the superficial mucosal or cutaneous lesions are not amenable for sampling [13, 14]. The diagnostic sensitivity of TBB in the diagnosis of a broad spectrum of interstitial lung diseases (ILDs) ranges from 29 to 79% [15–19]. The British Thoracic Society Sarcoidosis Registry data has previously showed that transbronchial biopsies have lesser diagnostic yield than EBUS-TBNA [20].

Bronchoalveolar lavage findings supportive of sarcoidosis include predominant lymphocytosis on differential cell count analysis along with CD4/CD8 lymphocyte ratio of more than 1. Müller-Quernheim et al. demonstrated that inflammation is compartmentalized in sarcoidosis resulting in lymphocyte abundance in the involved organs [21]. In a study by Prasse et al., patients with sarcoidosis had higher expression of IL2, IFN gamma, and TNF alpha [22]. Furthermore, Tanriverdi et al. showed that high CD4/CD8 ratio, though specific is not a sensitive test for the diagnosis of sarcoidosis, and therefore, it does require clinico-radiological and pathological correlation [23]. BAL lymphocytosis of ≥40% in the appropriate clinical context would support the diagnosis of hypersensitivity pneumonitis or cellular nonspecific interstitial pneumonia (NSIP) over sarcoidosis [24]. However, bronchoalveolar lavage findings in isolation are unlikely to help establish the diagnosis of sarcoidosis.

2.2.2 Endobronchial ultrasound-guided transbronchial needle aspiration (EBUS-TBNA)

EBUS-TBNA has been significant in the diagnostic pathway of sarcoidosis and has obviated the need for a TBB (in most cases where mediastinal adenopathy is present) with associated risk of pneumothorax. EBUS-TBNA is a safe minimally invasive option and is the preferred diagnostic procedure before surgical techniques such as mediastinoscopy are considered for sampling mediastinal nodes [25].

Kitamura et al. demonstrated a sensitivity of 87.5% for combined cytological and histological examination [26]. A prospective study by Oki et al. compared the diagnostic yield of EBUS-TBNA and TBLB through a flexible bronchoscope in patients with stage I and II of sarcoidosis [27]. The diagnostic yield was 94% (stage I, 97%; stage II, 88%) and 37% (stage I, 31%; stage II, 50%), respectively; the complications such as pneumothorax and moderate bleeding were noted in patients, who underwent TBLB, albeit one case of pneumothorax and three cases of moderate bleeding among a total of 62 patients were seen.

A randomized controlled trial evaluated the use of endosonographic nodal aspiration against bronchoscopic biopsy, among patients with suspected stage I/II pulmonary sarcoidosis [28]. The diagnostic yield to detect granulomas for endosonography was 80% (95% CI, 73–86%), in comparison to 53% (95% CI, 45–61%) for bronchoscopy cohort ($P < 0.001$), suggesting a significantly higher diagnostic yield with endosonographic procedures. On the other hand, a randomized controlled trial by Gupta et al. showed that the diagnostic yield in sarcoidosis by conventional TBNA along with endobronchial biopsy (EBB) and TBLB is similar to EBUS-TBNA with TBLB [29].

The diagnostic accuracy of EBUS-TBNA with rapid on-site evaluation (ROSE) was compared to the final cytological assessment and to TBLB and EBB in a prospective study, and it showed that sensitivity for EBUS-TBNA with ROSE was 87.8% (specificity 91%, positive predictive value 97.7%) and concluded that it should be considered as first-line investigation for the evaluation of mediastinal adenopathy [30].

In patients with predominant mediastinal and/or intra-abdominal lymph nodes, which is not amenable for EBUS procedure, endoscopic ultrasound-guided fine aspiration (EUS-FNA) can be a potential option; Michael et al. demonstrated in a retrospective study that [31] EUS-FNA was able to diagnose sarcoidosis in 86% of cases ($n = 18$ of 21) and was able to rule out recurrence of malignancy in 75% (three out of four cases).

2.2.3 Transbronchial lung cryobiopsy (TBLC)

Transbronchial lung cryobiopsy is currently being increasingly considered as a diagnostic tool in ILD. The procedure requires general anesthesia and fluoroscopic guidance for sampling with a cryoprobe [32]. In a retrospective study by Jacob et al., they were able to demonstrate a diagnostic yield of up to 92.6% on a small sample size in the study [33]. The main advantage of TBLC is related to larger biopsy sample in comparison to traditional transbronchial biopsy with associated crushing artifact of the sample. However, TBLC has the limitations related to training and the need for general anesthesia. Moreover, there is a significant risk of complications including pneumothorax and bleeding ranging from 9 to 10% and from 14 to 20%, respectively [34].

Hagmeyer et al. demonstrated that the risk of severe complications can be reduced from 84 to 14% by technical modification of this procedure. Hence, it may prove to be a useful step before consideration of surgical lung biopsy [35].

2.3 Ultrasound (US)-guided biopsy

The diagnostic workup for sarcoidosis should include the least invasive investigation at the outset of evaluation; thus, neck ultrasound may provide an ideal modality for that purpose. We have demonstrated that a core biopsy of cervical lymph nodes (ranging from 7 to 14 mm in diameter), with no sonographic appearance of being marked was adequate to make a histological diagnosis of sarcoidosis [36]. In this retrospective analysis, we showed that if there were no suitable cervical lymph node for biopsy, an US evaluation and biopsy of abnormal parotid glands may help establish the diagnosis of sarcoidosis [36]. In view of the ease of this procedure and its cost-effectiveness (approximately £1000/= saving in comparison to EBUS-TBNA per patient in the UK), this could potentially be considered as a first-line investigation if appropriate expertise is available. Hence, it is proposed that the diagnostic algorithm as shown in **Figure 5** for the investigation of mediastinal lymphadenopathy should include US-guided core biopsy of cervical lymph nodes +/− parotid glands if deemed abnormal. We envisage that a prospective multicenter study of wider application of this technique would be desirable to generalize the use of this minimally invasive diagnostic modality.

2.4 Surgical techniques: cervical mediastinoscopy and video-assisted thoracoscopy (VATS)

2.4.1 Cervical mediastinoscopy

Cervical mediastinoscopy (CM) is one of the preferred surgical techniques to evaluate mediastinal lymphadenopathy. The procedure helps to obtain samples from paratracheal and subcarinal lymph nodes. Since the advent of EBUS-TBNA, EUS-FNA, and PET-CT, the frequency of mediastinoscopy as a diagnostic procedure has declined significantly. Moreover, it is reserved when the above techniques have been inconclusive or not feasible due to the location of the enlarged lymph node.

Onat et al. reported the safety of CM and demonstrated that it is a reliable method, in the evaluation of mediastinal lymphadenopathy [37]. In a meta-analysis by Agarwal et al., they reported a diagnostic yield between 82 and 97% for cervical mediastinoscopy [38].

2.4.2 Video-assisted thoracoscopic surgery (VATS)

VATS biopsy should be considered when there is difficulty in establishing the diagnosis with other less invasive options especially if a specific histological diagnosis would help the prognosis or treatment [39]. The diagnostic yield, sensitivity,

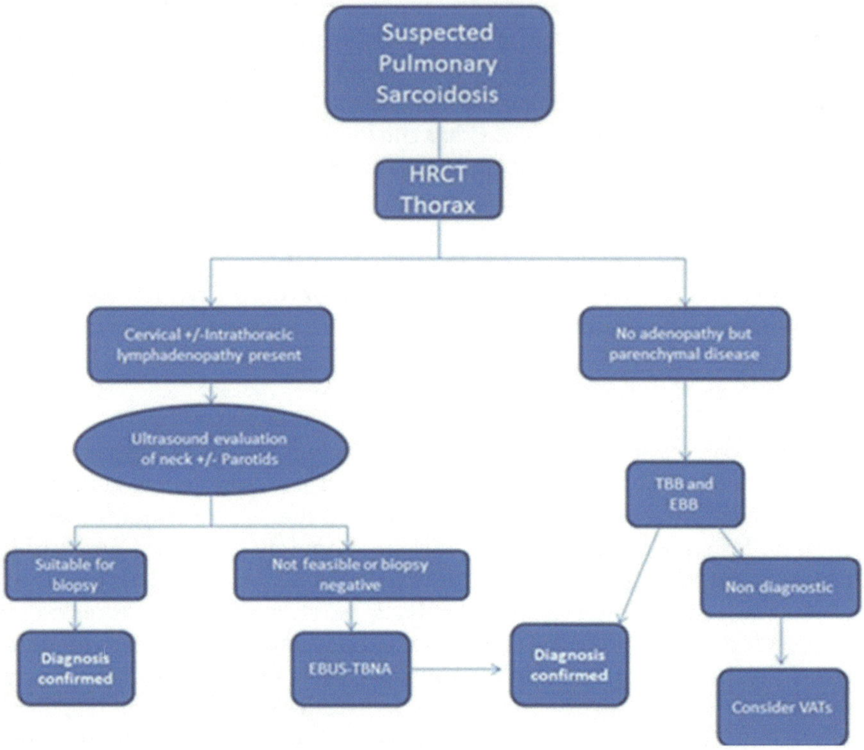

Figure 5.
Diagnostic approach in suspected pulmonary sarcoidosis. EBUS-TBNA, endobronchial ultrasound-guided transbronchial needle aspiration; TBB, transbronchial biopsy; EBB, endobronchial biopsy; VATS, video-assisted thoracoscopic biopsy [36].

and specificity of VATS reported in a meta-analysis were 92.7% (87.6–95.8%), 91% (89–92%), and 58% (31–81%), respectively [40]. VATS procedures have the advantage of technically enabling multilobed biopsies in comparison to open lung biopsy [41]. Currently, mini-VATS is also being increasingly considered given the less postoperative complications and decreased length of hospital stay [42, 43]. VATS procedure should be done by experienced thoracic surgeons, as there is a potential need for mini-thoracotomy in 25% of cases, to obtain adequate tissue for diagnosis [44]. Furthermore, there is a mortality rate of approximately 2% at 30 days associated with this surgical procedure as demonstrated by a meta-analysis conducted by Wallis et al. [45].

3. Conclusion

Sarcoidosis presents as a diagnostic dilemma in a number of medical specialties ranging from pulmonology, general internal medicine, rheumatology, and oncology to name a few. The advent of ultrasound-guided techniques (EBUS-TBNA, EUS-TBNA, and US-guided core biopsy of neck nodes) has significantly reduce the frequency of more invasive diagnostic procedures such as mediastinoscopy and surgical lung biopsies (both open and VATS biopsies). Moreover, TBB is rarely required to sample the lung parenchyma as the diagnostic yield of alternative procedures, with much less associated risk of pneumothorax (EBUS, EUS and US-guided core biopsy of neck nodes), is very high in appropriate clinical context. TBLC may be a newer diagnostic intervention being utilized in selected centers for histological assessment of ILDs, but its role in the diagnostic pathway is uncertain at present. However, future studies may shed light on its value in the diagnostic pathway of ILD. It is proposed that expertise for US-guided neck node core biopsy would be an important adjunct in the armory of interventional radiologists skill sets and has the potential to be a safe and cost-effective procedure in suspected pulmonary sarcoidosis. Furthermore, learning this technique to sample near normal-sized lymph nodes would be appropriate in minimizing bronchoscopic procedures, preventing significantly higher morbidity.

Acknowledgements

We thank Mr. John Hudson, the librarian at the New Cross Hospital, for his help with the literature review for this chapter.

Conflict of interest

The authors declare no conflict of interest in relation to this manuscript.

Author details

Rajarajan Anandavelu and Ahmed Fahim*
New Cross Hospital, Wolverhampton, UK

*Address all correspondence to: ahmedfahim@doctors.org.uk

References

[1] Calandriello L, Walsh SLF. Imaging for sarcoidosis. Seminars in Respiratory and Critical Care Medicine. 2017;**38**(4):417-436

[2] Drent M, De Vries J, Lenters M, Lamers RJ, Rothkranz-Kos S, Wouters EF, et al. Sarcoidosis: Assessment of disease severity using HRCT. European Radiology. 2003;**13**(11):2462-2471

[3] Ganeshan D, Menias CO, Lubner MG, Pickhardt PJ, Sandrasegaran K, Bhalla S. Sarcoidosis from head to toe: What the radiologist needs to know. Radiographics. 2018;**38**(4):1180-1200

[4] De Boer S, Milne DG, Zeng I, Wilsher ML. Does CT scanning predict the likelihood of a positive transbronchial biopsy in sarcoidosis? Thorax. 2009;**64**(5):436-439

[5] Mostard RL, van Kroonenburgh MJ, Drent M. The role of the PET scan in the management of sarcoidosis. Current Opinion in Pulmonary Medicine. 2013;**19**(5):538-544

[6] Yakar A, Yakar F, Sezer M, Bayram M, Erdogan EB, Ozkan D, et al. Use of PET-CT for the assessment of treatment results in patients with sarcoidosis. Wiener Klinische Wochenschrift. 2015;**127**(7-8):274-282

[7] Keijsers RG, Verzijlbergen EJ, van den Bosch JM, Zanen P, van de Garde EM, Oyen WJ, et al. 18F-FDG PET as a predictor of pulmonary function in sarcoidosis. Sarcoidosis, Vasculitis, and Diffuse Lung Diseases. 2011;**28**(2):123-129

[8] Maturu VN, Rayamajhi SJ, Agarwal R, Aggarwal AN, Gupta D, Mittal BR. Role of serial F-18 FDG PET/CT scans in assessing treatment response and predicting relapses in patients with symptomatic sarcoidosis. Sarcoidosis, Vasculitis, and Diffuse Lung Diseases. 2016;**33**(4):372-380

[9] Teirstein AS, Machac J, Almeida O, Lu P, Padilla ML, Iannuzzi MC. Results of 188 whole-body fluorodeoxyglucose positron emission tomography scans in 137 patients with sarcoidosis. Chest. 2007;**132**(6):1949-1953

[10] Yu C, Xia X, Qin C, Sun X, Zhang Y, Lan X. Is SUVmax helpful in the differential diagnosis of enlarged mediastinal lymph nodes? A Pilot Study. Contrast Media & Molecular Imaging. 2018;**2018**:3417190

[11] Viles-Gonzalez JF, Pastori L, Fischer A, Wisnivesky JP, Goldman MG, Mehta D. Supraventricular arrhythmias in patients with cardiac sarcoidosis prevalence, predictors, and clinical implications. Chest. 2013;**143**(4):1085-1090

[12] Smedema JP, van Geuns RJ, Ector J, Heidbuchel H, Ainslie G, Crijns H. Right ventricular involvement and the extent of left ventricular enhancement with magnetic resonance predict adverse outcome in pulmonary sarcoidosis. ESC Heart Failure. 2018;**5**(1):157-171

[13] Fahim A, Mann JS. Pulmonary sarcoidosis: Diagnostic and treatment update. Expert Review of Respiratory Medicine. 2014;**8**(4):493-501

[14] Hsu RM, Connors AF Jr, Tomashefski JF Jr. Histologic, microbiologic, and clinical correlates of the diagnosis of sarcoidosis by transbronchial biopsy. Archives of Pathology & Laboratory Medicine. 1996;**120**(4):364-368

[15] Shorr AF, Torrington KG, Hnatiuk OW. Endobronchial biopsy for sarcoidosis: A prospective study. Chest. 2001;**120**(1):109-114

[16] Mitchell DM, Mitchell DN, Collins JV, Emerson CJ. Transbronchial lung biopsy through fibreoptic bronchoscope in diagnosis of sarcoidosis. British Medical Journal. 1980;**280**(6215):679-681

[17] Haponik EF, Summer WR, Terry PB, Wang KP. Clinical decision making with transbronchial lung biopsies. The value of nonspecific histologic examination. The American Review of Respiratory Disease. 1982;**125**(5):524-529

[18] Wall CP, Gaensler EA, Carrington CB, Hayes JA. Comparison of transbronchial and open biopsies in chronic infiltrative lung diseases. The American Review of Respiratory Disease. 1981;**123**(3):280-285

[19] Poletti V, Patelli M, Ferracini R, Simonetti M, Spiga L. Transbronchial lung biopsy in infiltrative lung disease. The importance of the pathologic approach. Sarcoidosis. 1988;**5**(1):43-50

[20] Thillai M, Chang W, Chaudhuri N, Forrest I, Ho LP, Lines S, et al. Sarcoidosis in the UK: Insights from British Thoracic Society registry data. BMJ Open Respiratory Research. 2019;**6**(1):e000357

[21] Muller-Quernheim J, Saltini C, Sondermeyer P, Crystal RG. Compartmentalized activation of the interleukin 2 gene by lung T lymphocytes in active pulmonary sarcoidosis. Journal of Immunology. 1986;**137**(11):3475-3483

[22] Prasse A, Georges CG, Biller H, Hamm H, Matthys H, Luttmann W, et al. Th1 cytokine pattern in sarcoidosis is expressed by bronchoalveolar CD4+ and CD8+ T cells. Clinical and Experimental Immunology. 2000;**122**(2):241-248

[23] Tanriverdi H, Erboy F, Altinsoy B, Uygur F, Arasli M, Ozel Tekin I, et al. Bronchoalveolar lavage fluid characteristics of patients with sarcoidosis and nonsarcoidosis interstitial lung diseases: Ten-year experience of a single center in Turkey. Iranian Red Crescent Medical Journal. 2015;**17**(10):e31103

[24] Meyer KC, Raghu G, Baughman RP, Brown KK, Costabel U, du Bois RM, et al. An official American Thoracic Society clinical practice guideline: The clinical utility of bronchoalveolar lavage cellular analysis in interstitial lung disease. American Journal of Respiratory and Critical Care Medicine. 2012;**185**(9):1004-1014

[25] Garwood S, Judson MA, Silvestri G, Hoda R, Fraig M, Doelken P. Endobronchial ultrasound for the diagnosis of pulmonary sarcoidosis. Chest. 2007;**132**(4): 1298-1304

[26] Kitamura A, Takiguchi Y, Kurosu K, Takigawa N, Saegusa F, Hiroshima K, et al. Feasibility of cytological diagnosis of sarcoidosis with endobronchial US-guided transbronchial aspiration. Sarcoidosis, Vasculitis, and Diffuse Lung Diseases. 2012;**29**(2):82-89

[27] Oki M, Saka H, Kitagawa C, Kogure Y, Murata N, Ichihara S, et al. Prospective study of endobronchial ultrasound-guided transbronchial needle aspiration of lymph nodes versus transbronchial lung biopsy of lung tissue for diagnosis of sarcoidosis. The Journal of Thoracic and Cardiovascular Surgery. 2012;**143**(6):1324-1329

[28] Von Bartheld MB, Dekkers OM, Szlubowski A, Eberhardt R, Herth FJ, in 't Veen JC, et al. Endosonography vs conventional bronchoscopy for the diagnosis of sarcoidosis: The GRANULOMA randomized clinical trial. Journal of the American Medical Association. 2013;**309**(23):2457-2464

[29] Gupta D, Dadhwal DS, Agarwal R, Gupta N, Bal A, Aggarwal AN.

Endobronchial ultrasound-guided transbronchial needle aspiration vs conventional transbronchial needle aspiration in the diagnosis of sarcoidosis. Chest. 2014;**146**(3):547-556

[30] Plit ML, Havryk AP, Hodgson A, James D, Field A, Carbone S, et al. Rapid cytological analysis of endobronchial ultrasound-guided aspirates in sarcoidosis. The European Respiratory Journal. 2013;**42**(5):1302-1308

[31] Michael H, Ho S, Pollack B, Gupta M, Gress F. Diagnosis of intra-abdominal and mediastinal sarcoidosis with EUS-guided FNA. Gastrointestinal Endoscopy. 2008;**67**(1):28-34

[32] Pedro C, Melo N, Novais EBH, Magalhaes A, Fernandes G, Martins N, et al. Role of bronchoscopic techniques in the diagnosis of thoracic sarcoidosis. Journal of Clinical Medicine. 2019;**8**(9):1327. DOI: 10.3390/jcm8091327

[33] Jacob M, Bastos HN, Mota PC, Melo N, Cunha R, Pereira JM, et al. Diagnostic yield and safety of transbronchial cryobiopsy in sarcoidosis. ERJ Open Research. 2019;**5**(4):00203-2019. DOI: 10.1183/23120541.00203-2019

[34] Shafiq M, Lee H, Yarmus L, Feller-Kopman D. Recent advances in interventional pulmonology. Annals of the American Thoracic Society. 2019;**16**(7):786-796

[35] Hagmeyer L, Theegarten D, Wohlschlager J, Hager T, Treml M, Herkenrath SD, et al. Transbronchial cryobiopsy in fibrosing interstitial lung disease: Modifications of the procedure lead to risk reduction. Thorax. 2019;**74**(7):711-714

[36] Fahim A, Qasim MM, Rosewarne D. Neck as mediastinal extension: Diagnosis of sarcoidosis by core biopsy of cervical lymph nodes. The Clinical Respiratory Journal. 2020;**14**(1):16-20. DOI: 10.1111/crj.13094

[37] Onat S, Ates G, Avci A, Yildiz T, Birak A, Akgul Ozmen C, et al. The role of mediastinoscopy in the diagnosis of non-lung cancer diseases. Therapeutics and Clinical Risk Management. 2017;**13**:939-943

[38] Agarwal R, Srinivasan A, Aggarwal AN, Gupta D. Efficacy and safety of convex probe EBUS-TBNA in sarcoidosis: A systematic review and meta-analysis. Respiratory Medicine. 2012;**106**(6):883-892

[39] Deconinck B, Verschakelen J, Coolen J, Verbeken E, Verleden G, Wuyts W. Diagnostic workup for diffuse parenchymal lung disease: Schematic flowchart, literature review, and pitfalls. Lung. 2013;**191**(1):19-25

[40] Iftikhar IH, Alghothani L, Sardi A, Berkowitz D, Musani AI. Transbronchial lung cryobiopsy and video-assisted thoracoscopic lung biopsy in the diagnosis of diffuse parenchymal lung disease. A meta-analysis of diagnostic test accuracy. Annals of the American Thoracic Society. 2017;**14**(7):1197-1211

[41] Bradley B, Branley HM, Egan JJ, Greaves MS, Hansell DM, Harrison NK, et al. Interstitial lung disease guideline: The British Thoracic Society in collaboration with the Thoracic Society of Australia and New Zealand and the Irish Thoracic Society. Thorax. 2008;**63**(Suppl 5):v1-v58

[42] Jeon CS, Yoon DW, Moon SM, Shin S, Cho JH, Lee SM, et al. Non-intubated video-assisted thoracoscopic lung biopsy for interstitial lung disease: A single-center experience. Journal of Thoracic Disease. 2018;**10**(6):3262-3268

[43] Massone PP, Lequaglie C, Magnani B, Ferro F, Cataldo I. The real impact and usefulness of video-assisted

thoracoscopic surgery in the diagnosis and therapy of clinical lymphadenopathies of the mediastinum. Annals of Surgical Oncology. 2003;**10**(10):1197-1202

[44] Hsu CP, Hanke I, Douglas JM Jr. Diagnostic video-assisted thoracoscopic procedures. Annals of Surgery. 1995;**222**(5):626-631

[45] Wallis A, Spinks K. The diagnosis and management of interstitial lung diseases. BMJ. 2015;**350**:h2072

Chapter 3

Early Diagnosis of Sarcoidosis

Marica Tina Maccarone

Abstract

Sarcoidosis is a rare unknown etiology multisystem inflammatory disease in which noncaseating granulomas (a collection of inflammatory cells) forms and growth in various organs, involving predominantly lungs, intrathoracic lymph node, skin, and eyes. Most commonly, affecting patients between 20 and 40 years old of age, although could be observed at any age (female predominance; rare in Asians). The areas of the body usually affected by sarcoidosis are lungs, skin, or lymph nodes; pulmonary and mediastinal involvement is seen in over 90% of patients. Less commonly eyes, liver, heart, and brain are involved. Any organ, however, can be affected. Early diagnosis of sarcoidosis can be difficult due to few signs and symptoms in its early stages, and when disease does occur, it may mimic other pathologies, and it is achieved through chest X-ray, computed tomography (CT)-high resolution CT (HRCT), gallium scans. Fluoro-deoxy glucose-positron emission tomography (FDG-PET) is another useful tool to assess the extent of disease and has a potential to evaluate the clinical management of patients responding or not to the treatment. Imaging gives, moreover, an important contribution to the evaluation of prognosis and follow-up.

Keywords: sarcoidosis, diagnosis, early diagnosis, chest X-ray, computed tomography (CT)-high resolution CT (HRCT), gallium scans, fluoro-deoxy glucose-positron emission tomography (FDG-PET)

1. Introduction

Sarcoidosis is a rare unknown etiology multiorgan granulomatous disease. The most affected organs by the pathology are the lungs, skin, or lymph nodes (especially intrathoracic lymph nodes). Less commonly are involved eyes, liver, heart, and brain, in a percentage ranging between 25 and 50%. Any organ, however, can be involved by sarcoidosis [1].

Signs and symptoms depend on which organs are affected and the presentation varies with the extent and severity of organ involvement [2].

The first state is *asymptomatic phase* (incidentally detected on chest imaging), approximately in 5% of patients. Then, *systemic complaints* are possible, which manifest itself with fever and anorexia (about 45% of cases). The most common condition (about 50% of cases) is *pulmonary complaints* with clinical presentation of dyspnea on exertion, cough, chest pain, and rarely hemoptysis. Pulmonary findings usually are normal but crackles may be audible; furthermore in a little part of patients exertional oxygen desaturation may be present [2].

Another possible clinical presentation is *Löfgren syndrome*, which consists in fever, bilateral hilar lymphadenopathy, erythema nodosum (an acute, nodular, cutaneous rash), and arthritis with polyarthralgias and is common in Scandinavian patients, but quite uncommon in African-American and Japanese patients. *Cutaneous involvement* may be present not only with erythema nodosum associated with Löfgren syndrome, but also with lupus pernio, violaceous rash on the cheeks or nose (quite common) and maculopapular plaques (quite uncommon) [2].

Ocular involvement is also possible, which may lead to blindness for untreated anterior or (most frequent) posterior granulomatous uveitis, conjunctival lesions and scleral plaques.

Other uncommon possible manifestations are [2] *nervous system involvement* with lymphocytic meningitis (rare), cranial nerve palsies, hypothalamic/pituitary dysfunction (rare) with diabetes insipidus and myelopathy; *heart failure* from cardiomyopathy (rare) or heart block and sudden death; *osseous involvement* with arthritic syndromes; *blood abnormalities*: anemia, leukopenia, thrombocytopenia and hemolytic anemia with or without splenomegaly (without splenomegaly may reflect bone marrow involvement); *gastrointestinal and genitourinary involvement* (rare): hepatomegaly, cholestasis, portal hypertension, Crohn's disease, pancreatic involvement, nephrocalcinosis, vulva itchiness and male infertility (rare); *exocrine and endocrine manifestations* with hyperprolactinemia, amenorrhea, galactorrhea, or nonpuerperal mastitis in women; hypercalciuria and hypercalcemia likely result from the increased 1,25-dihydroxy vitamin D production (rare) [2].

2. Diagnosis

The diagnosis is based on clinical and imaging features, histological confirmation, and exclusion of other diseases that can create similar histopathological and clinical findings.

Imaging is mandatory for diagnosis of sarcoidosis and includes as follows:

- chest radiography (is fundamental for a first evaluation);
- routine chest computed tomography (CT), usually high-resolution CT (HRCT) scanning of the chest [2] (has a significantly superior detection rate to chest X-ray for mediastinal and pulmonary parenchymal changes and is also useful to identify active alveolitis or fibrosis), and the agreement between findings and biopsy yield [2]; and
- fluoro-deoxy glucose-positron emission tomography (FDG-PET) combined with CT-scan (is fundamental to determinte the extent of organ involvement and the disease activity and to evaluate the response to pharmacological therapy) [3].

2.1 Chest X-rays and HRCT scan

A correct staging of pulmonary sarcoidosis based on radiological stage of the disease is necessary to evaluate the sarcoidosis prognosis [1]. Particularly, there are five radiologic stages (forms) of intrathoracic sarcoidosis on chest radiography [2–4] as follows:

- Stage 0: normal chest radiographic findings;
- Stage I: bilateral mediastinal lymphadenopathy (hilar lymphadenopathy);

- Stage II: bilateral mediastinal lymphadenopathy (hilar lymphadenopathy) and infiltrates with parenchymal lesion;
- Stage III: infiltrates alone, parenchymal disease only; and
- Stage IV: pulmonary fibrosis.

HRCT, however, is more accurate in identifying the different manifestations of pulmonary sarcoidosis as well its complications, but we are still searching for an accepted HRCT scoring system.

Main findings of HRCT sarcoidosis are as follows:

- hilar and/or mediastinal lymph node enlargement (sometimes with calcifications), classically bilateral hilar and right paratracheal nodal enlargement (Garland triad); left paratracheal and aortopulmonary nodes can be also enlarged. Atypical pattern of nodal enlargement can be observed in patients older than 50 years old of age;
- pulmonary interstitial nodules (micro or macronodules) in a perilymphatic distribution;
- thickening of the peribronchovascular interstitium;
- pulmonary ground glass opacity;
- consolidation or large nodular opacities;
- coarse linear opacities, interlobular septal thickening, honeycombing, and cysts;
- architectural distortion, superior hilar retraction, or traction bronchiectasis; and
- pulmonary fibrosis (Stage IV) with linear bands of fibrosis from hila to all directions with distortion of normal lung architecture; honeycombing is rare, only in patients with severe fibrosis, mainly in the middle and upper lung zones and with subpleural involvement.

Pleural disease is rare and may be observed when disease is extensive.

The diagnosis of pulmonary sarcoidosis requires a compatible clinical picture supported by radiologic (X-rays chest and/or HRCT of lungs) and pathologic data (pulmonary functional tests and laboratory tests). But for a certain diagnosis, biopsy is required in most cases, and endobronchial biopsy via bronchoscopy is often performed; its results may be positive even in patients with normal chest radiographs. The central histologic finding is the presence of noncaseating granulomas with special stains negative for fungi and mycobacteria [2].

2.2 Cardiopulmonary and laboratory tests

Pulmonary function tests are also routinely used in sarcoidosis for early diagnosis and follow-up. They include the evaluation of forced vital capacity (FVC), forced expiratory volume in one second (FEV1), the total lung capacity determination (TLC), vital capacity (VC), residual volume (RV) associated with body plethysmography, and a carbon monoxide diffusion capacity test of the lungs for carbon monoxide (DLCO).

Sarcoidosis is commonly considered a restrictive disorder, but more recent studies are demonstrating some opposite results.

Restrictive disorders (infiltrative) are characterized by a reduction in lung volume, with difficult in taking air inside the lungs and decreased total lung capacity. Other restrictive disorders are chest wall disorders (neuromuscular, e.g., polio, kyphoscoliosis, pleural disease, and severe obesity); chronic interstitial and infiltrative disease (pulmonary fibrosis, pneumoconioses, granulomatous diseases, pulmonary eosinophilia, and pulmonary alveolar proteinosis); Acute diseases (ARDS and infections).

Typical symptoms are dyspnea, tachypnea, end inspiratory crackles without airway obstruction, honey-comb lung, secondary pulmonary hypertension, and cor pulmonale.

In restrictive pulmonary disease, lung volume is decrease, but flow rate is normal as follows:

- TLC decrease;
- RV decrease;
- FEV1 decrease;
- FVC decrease;
- FEV1/VC is equal to or more than 70%;
- DLCO decrease; and
- compliance decrease.

Usually, a significant correlation between radiological stage and pulmonary function tests is found.

Cardiopulmonary exercise testing (CPET) is another useful tool to identify and quantify the extent of pulmonary involvement and also may suggest cardiac involvement that otherwise is not evident [2]. It provides an integrative assessment of involving the pulmonary, cardiovascular, muscular, and cellular oxidative systems and involves measurements of gas exchange as follows:

- primarily oxygen uptake (VO_2): VO_2 at maximal exercise (peak VO_2) is considered the best index of aerobic capacity and cardiorespiratory function;
- carbon dioxide output (VCO_2);
- minute ventilation; and
- anaerobic threshold (lactic acid).

In patients who have normal gas exchange at rest, CPET unmasks the gas exchange abnormalities.

Laboratory tests can identify some serum abnormalities as high blood calcium with a normal parathyroid hormone level and hypercalciuria, or elevated levels of angiotensin converting enzyme (ACE) in the blood [1].

2.3 FDG-PET

FDG-PET is a metabolic imaging technique and provides an insight into metabolism of this disease. It relies on the principle of increased accumulation and metabolism of glucose by the malignant or inflammatory areas. FDG is a radioactive analog of glucose that enters cells through the same receptors that are involved in glucose uptake and gets converted into FDG 6 phosphate by the enzyme hexokinase, similar to glucose metabolism by the glycolytic pathway. FDG 6 phosphate is not metabolized further and gets entrapped in the cell. Tissues with high glucose metabolism such as brain tissue gray matter, cancer cells, and inflammatory changes show increased fluorine – 18 fluorodeoxyglucose ((18) F-FDG) accumulation on PET imaging.

As a key component of the inflammatory process, inflammatory cells consume glucose at a much higher level than peripheral noninflammatory cells, leading to higher glucose metabolism and increased uptake of (18) F-FDG within inflammatory foci. Therefore, the level of FDG uptake is proportional to the level of glycolysis in the tissue. This explains the mechanism of increased uptake of FDG in malignancy, inflammatory, and infectious processes [3].

The role of fluoro-deoxy glucose-positron emission tomography (FDG-PET) scanning in assessing the extent of disease spread or metastasis and its utility in assessing response to treatment in the form of chemotherapy or radiotherapy is well defined in many neoplastic conditions, and its utility has also been recognized in certain inflammatory conditions, like sarcoidosis.

During the last years, FDG-PET imaging has been shown to have a central role to detect inflammation activity and has become a novel fundamental tool, playing also an increasingly important role in the management of patients with any inflammatory conditions. FDG-PET can afford precious information in patients with pulmonary and extrapulmonary sarcoidosis and has become a centerpiece for testing the efficacy of different therapies [5]. In difficult clinical cases, it can also be useful to plan the site of biopsy in order to determinate a histopathological diagnosis.

A combined modality using FDG-PET and CT scanning (FDG-PET/CT) has been found to be more sensitive than PET in diagnosing. FDG-PET and a combination of this procedure with computed tomography scanning (FDG-PET/CT) has gained prominent attention in patients with sarcoidosis over the last two decades as a means to assess disease activity and response to therapy. Radionuclide imaging techniques have increasingly been used in the evaluation of organ involvement in sarcoidosis. F-FDG-PET/CT scanning has received increasing attention in last several years [3].

The usefulness of F-FDG-PET/CT is to identify the disease activity and the extent of organ involvement in patients affected by sarcoidosis; F-FDG-PET/CT is still useful to determinate its utility in the evaluation of response to drug treatment, comparing the agreement between clinical, radiological (with chest radiography and/or HRCT of lungs), and metabolic indices (FDG-PET/CT) of disease activity.

Monitoring disease activity in sarcoidosis still remains a clinical goal as there is no gold standard. The term "activity" in sarcoidosis means ongoing inflammation that necessitates appropriate drug therapy [3]. PET imaging is a new tool to assess the metabolic activity, but there is still limited data on the role of serial PET scans in monitoring the sarcoidosis activity [6].

Conventional imaging techniques used in sarcoidosis are chest radiography and CT. Even though chest radiography and HR-CT are still the fundamental for diagnosing pulmonary involvement, F- FDG PET appears to be superior to both techniques to identify active sites of disease. F- FDG- PET also correlates well with serum biomarkers, such as soluble interleukin-2 receptor in symptomatic patients, and in lung parenchyma correlates with decrease of lung function values over time. Moreover F-FDG-PET even visualizes active lesions (in pulmonary and extrapulmonary sites) in the context of normal serum biomarkers. Also in cardiac involvement in sarcoidosis, FDG-PET is a promising tool associated or complementary to magnetic resonance imaging, especially in planning treatment [7].

Magnetic resonance imaging (MRI) is the main imaging method for diagnosis and follow-up of neurosarcoidosis and for evaluation of cardiac involvement. However, these mentioned methods are unable to identify active inflammation; instead, FDG-PET/CT has an important advantage in the detection of reversible, inflammatory, active granulomatous disease in patients with sarcoidosis [8].

PET provides high-resolution three-dimensional images of the whole body that facilitates precise localization of abnormalities. Localization is enhanced with PET/CT. Fluorodeoxyglucose is extremely sensitive with a high negative predictive value; however, the limiting factor of the test is specificity [9, 10]. (18) F-FDG PET/CT allows to obtain a complete morphofunctional cartography of inflammatory active localizations and to follow treatment efficacy in patients with sarcoidosis, particularly in atypical, complex, and multisystemic forms.

Disseminated lesions should alert clinician to consider sarcoidosis-lymphoma syndrome (SLS) or tuberculosis in the differential diagnosis. However, histological confirmation with biopsy will be required in such complex cases.

2.3.1 Pulmonary sarcoidosis

Pulmonary sarcoidosis is the main localization site in the majority of patients (>90% cases) typically with bilateral mediastinal (hilar) lymphadenopathy diagnosed on chest radiography; and its severity ranges from asymptomatic involvement of mediastinal lymph nodes (mostly hilar) to progressive pulmonary fibrosis and chronic respiratory failure that is unresponsive to therapy. The most common clinical presentations of pulmonary involvement are cough and dyspnea.

The diagnosis of pulmonary sarcoidosis requires a compatible clinical picture supported by radiologic (X-rays chest and/or HRCT of lungs) and pathologic data (pulmonary functional tests and laboratory tests). A recent innovation in diagnosing of pulmonary sarcoidosis is endobronchial ultrasound that increases the yield of transbronchial needle aspiration of hilar and/or mediastinal lymph nodes. F-FDG-PET is highly sensitive in detecting occult sites of disease and is very useful in guiding biopsies of these sites. A combined imaging modality using both FDG-PET and CT scan is more sensitive than PET alone and is now the main proceeding of care in patients needing biopsies of active lesions [11].

For staging of pulmonary disease on chest radiograph, Scadding stages (**Figure 1**) are still widely used depending on the presence of hilar lymph node enlargement and pulmonary opacities on chest radiography as follows:

- Stage 0: normal chest radiographic findings;
- Stage I: bilateral mediastinal lymphadenopathy (hilar lymphadenopathy);
- Stage II: bilateral mediastinal lymphadenopathy (hilar lymphadenopathy) and infiltrates with parenchymal lesion;
- Stage III: infiltrates alone, parenchymal disease only; and
- Stage IV: pulmonary fibrosis.

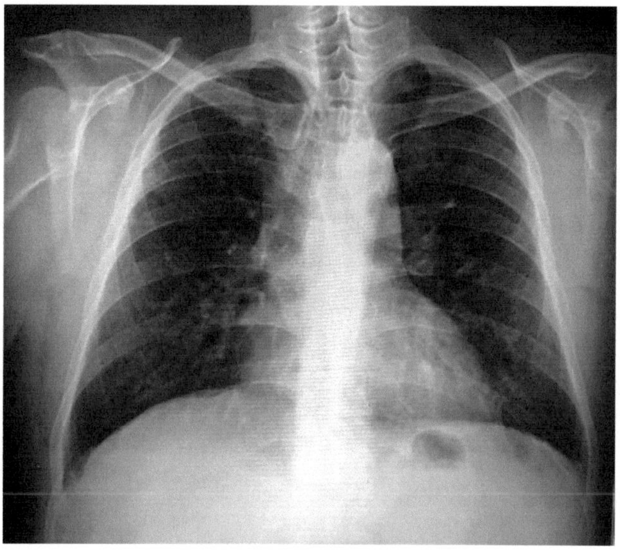

Figure 1.
Chest X-rays: reticulonodular pattern with perihilar distribution.

HRCT, however, is still the gold standard imaging modality for primary diagnosis of sarcoidosis and is more accurate than chest X-rays, which is the first imaging level, in identifying the different manifestations of pulmonary sarcoidosis as well its complications. F-FDG-PET, instead, is a new highly sensitive tool in detecting occult sites of disease at the chest CT scan.

HRCT most common signs are: micronodules (*miliary sarcoidosis*) and macronodules with perilymphatic distribution, for the most part, symmetrically in the middle zones of the lungs; rarely solitary opacity (*alveolar sarcoidosis*) and with a mass-like presentation (1–4 cm in diameter) may mimic consolidation containing air bronchograms, from confluence of many smaller nodules with irregular margins and presenting as *sarcoid galaxy sign* (mass-like region from confluence of numerous smaller granulomas with a central core and multiple peripheral nodules; central cavitation may occur, and the lesion can be surrounded by ground-glass opacity), more frequent in patients older than 50 years of age of presentation; linear opacities, mostly, in the upper and middle parts of the lungs, most common of stage II or III of disease; and ground glass opacities represent interstitial sarcoid granulomas under resolution rather than alveolitis, above all, located in the lower zones of the lungs [12] (**Figures 2–6**).

Functional imaging of sarcoidosis nowadays is performed with (18) F-FDG PET-CT, which improves anatomical localization of sites of abnormality and has a relatively short delay time between radiotracer injection and image acquisition. (18) F-FDG PET-CT can identify disease activity better than conventional makers in a large proportion of patients (very high sensitivity about 80–100%). In patients with positive HRCT but no parenchymal fluorodeoxyglucose F18 uptake, pay attention to initiation or intensification of immunosuppressive treatment [1, 13].

2.3.2 Cardiac sarcoidosis

Cardiac involvement in sarcoidosis is uncommon (5%) and is associated with very poor prognosis [1], because of many complications of cardiac as follows: ventricular tachycardia, conductional abnormalities, congestive heart failure, and sudden cardiac death. Moreover, cardiac sarcoidosis (CS) is an important prognostic factor in patients with this disease. However, early diagnosis of CS in still

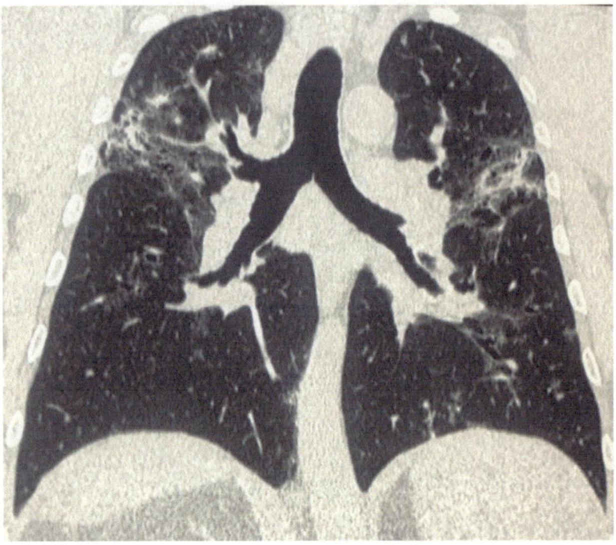

Figure 2.
HRCT: coarse linear opacities, architectural distortion, superior hilar retraction, and traction bronchiectasis.

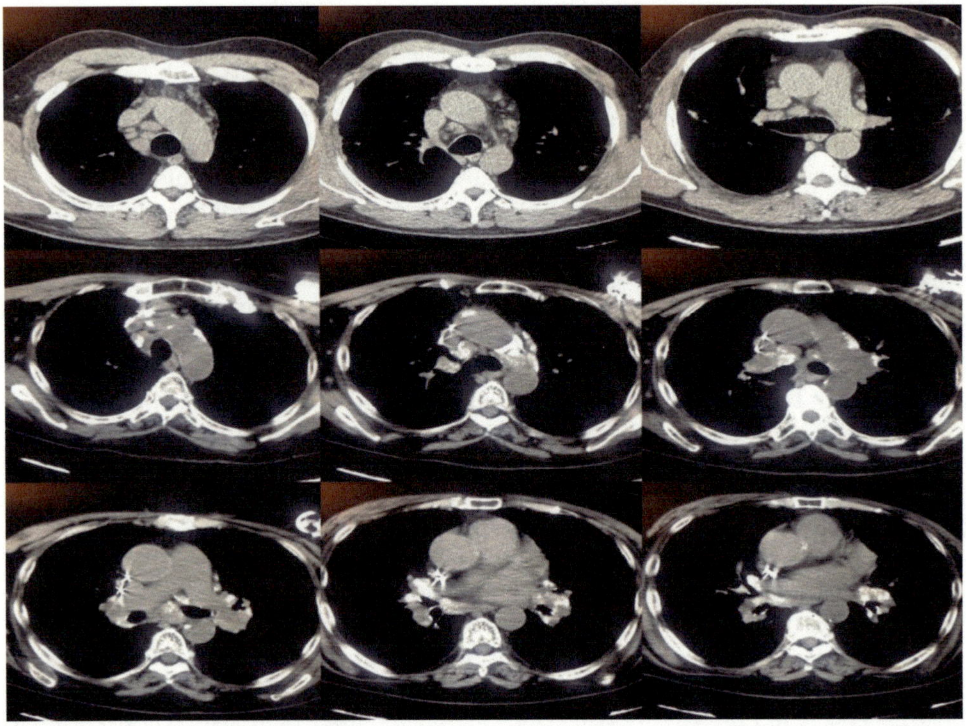

Figure 3.
HRCT: hilar and mediastinal lymph node enlargement, sometimes with calcification.

really difficult due to the nonspecific clinical manifestations of the disease, inhomogeneous myocardial involvement, and the limited diagnostic yield of diagnostic tests. Therefore, there are no standardized tests for the early diagnosis of cardiac sarcoidosis, although early detection of CS is very important for effective treatment. Besides a history and physical examination, electrocardiography (ECG) and transthoracic echocardiography are useful for cardiac evaluation.

Staging	Description
0	Absence of chest X-ray abnormalities
1	Bilateral hilar lymphadenopathy that may be accompanied by right paratracheal and aortopulmonary window adenopathy
2	Bilateral hilar lymphadenopathy and parenchymal infiltration with a bilateral symmetric micronodular or reticulonodular pattern with predominant perihilar distribution, in middle and upper lung fields
3	Parenchymal infiltration without hilar adenopathy
4	Fibrosis with evidence of reticular pattern with traction bronchiectasis, masses causing architectural distortions, or honeycomb cysts, predominantly in the upper fields

Figure 4.
Scadding stages for staging of pulmonary disease on chest X-rays.

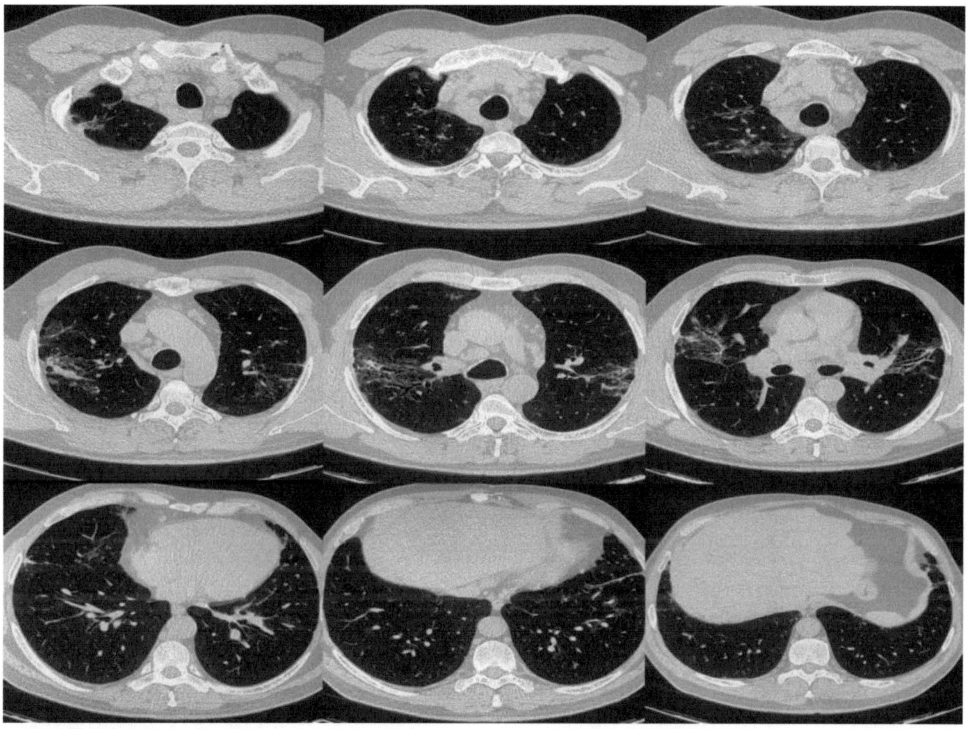

Figure 5.
HRCT: micronodules and macronodules with perilymphatic distribution, for the most part, symmetrically in the middle zones of the lungs; pulmonary ground glass areas; thickening of the peribronchovascular interstitium; coarse linear opacities and interlobular septal thickening; and architectural distortion, superior hilar retraction, and traction bronchiectasis.

CS can be diagnosed using (18) F-FDG-PET/CT (PET) and cardiovascular magnetic resonance (CMRI) that nowadays have been emerged as well for this purpose in recent clinical practice [1]. Imaging modalities that can both identify disease and predict response to therapy are supreme to improve management of cardiac sarcoidosis.

(18) F-FDG-PET has many practical advantages in identifying disease activity and monitoring treatment response in patients with CS [1]. In (18) F-FDG, increased uptake, indicating active inflammation, can be seen in CS in the myocardial wall [14, 15].

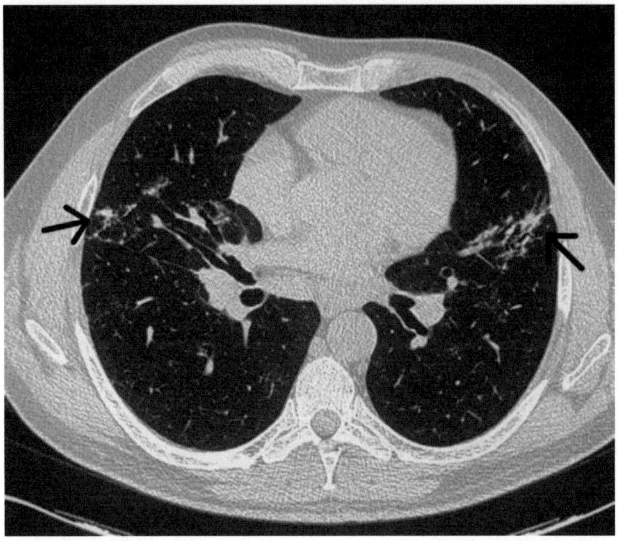

Figure 6.
Sarcoid galaxy sign: *mass-like region from confluence of numerous smaller granulomas with a central core and multiple peripheral nodules (arrows).*

Focal hypermetabolic activity or a focal increase of activity with a diffusely increased background on (18) F-FDG- PET is characteristic for cardiac sarcoidosis but this technique has some limitations. Normal myocardial cells use glucose as one of main energy substrates [14], and so physiologic (18) F-FDG uptake may be found in myocardium of healthy subjects; also papillary muscles and lateral wall of left ventricle may also show normal uptake of (18) F-FDG. Then, special patient preparation is, therefore, needed prior to F-FDG-PET scan in patients with sarcoidosis, with three different approaches: prolonged fasting, dietary modification with high-fat diet and i.v. administration of unfractionated heparin, trying to suppress (18) F-FDG uptake promoting fatty acid metabolism.

In cardiac sarcoidosis, the combined use of FDG-PET/CT and CMRI may provide optimal detection of the disease by enabling the differentiation between patients with active granulomatous inflammation and those with fibrous lesions. CMRI is a sensitive technique to assess the locations and extent of disease. Myocardial sarcoidosis may present on CMRI as segmental wall motion abnormality, focal wall thickening or thinning, or nodules with a patchy distribution [3].

On CMRI scan, in CS, we can find late gadolinium enhancement (LGE) related to the presence of fibrous granulomatous tissue, areas with an increased signal on T2-weighted sequences consistent with myocardial edema and with hypointensity suggesting fibrosis [10]. Recently, the value of LGE on CMRI, which allows visualization of even minute amounts of myocardial damage, has been emphasized in diagnosing CS, and it might be a promising tool for determining the prognosis of patients with biopsy-proven extracardiac sarcoidosis [1, 16].

However, it is not easy to differentiate between active and inactive sarcoidosis lesions, which is important for patient management. In addition, cardiac MRI is generally contraindicated in patients with pacemakers or implantable cardioverter defibrillators (ICDs).

2.3.3 Neurosarcoidosis

Nervous system involvement is not an uncommon manifestation of sarcoidosis and can be clinically symptomatic neurosarcoidosis, which occurs in 5–16% of patients with sarcoidosis, and subclinical neurosarcoidosis, with an incidence of subclinical disease that may be higher [17–19]. The neurological manifestations depend on the areas of the nervous system involved.

The most commonly involved part are cranial nerves, though any part of neuroaxis can be affected. The facial nerve is the most common cranial nerve involved presenting with facial palsy, and the second most common nerve affected is the optic nerve presenting with diplopia or impaired visual acuity [3, 19].

Neurosarcoidosis in the brain can present with leptomeningeal and intraparenchymal infiltration of granulomas resulting, for example, in cranial nerve palsies, basal meningitis, and endocrine dysfunction. It can cause also peripheral neuropathies (such as sensorimotor polyneuropathy, radiculopathy, and myopathy) [3]. For all of these reasons, neurosarcoidosis is an important cause of morbidity and mortality in patients with sarcoidosis.

Diagnosis and management of patients with neurosarcoidosis are still challenging because the gold standard is tissue-proven biopsy but, in most cases of nervous system involvement, it is really difficult to obtain [3, 18].

Contrast-enhanced MRI for the detection of intracranial and spinal cord lesions is the imaging modality of choice for evaluating neurosarcoidosis. However, the findings on MRI are often nonspecific.

In central nervous system (CNS) involvement, the hypointensity of signal of the dural and of parenchymal lesions in T2-weighted sequences is useful to identify sarcoidosis. Contrast-enhanced MRI is a sensitive tool in the detection of CNS inflammation but has a low specificity, making the correct diagnosis of neurosarcoidosis still a clinical challenge.

The most common imaging finding in T2-weighted sequences are hyperintense parenchymal lesions (gray matter) and in T1-weighted sequences, after intravascular administration of contrast agents, are meningeal enhancement (basilar meningitis involving of cranial nerves is thought to be a common phenomenon), and swelling and/or enhancement of optic nerves or chiasm maybe with associated visual loss. Other imaging presentations include intracranial masses simulating neoplasms and vasculitic infarcts. Moreover, in a small part of cases, brain MRI can be normal. Cervical or thoracolumbar spine abnormalities, such as spinal cord swelling, meningeal enhancement, and parenchymal contrast enhancing lesions, can also be detected [20].

Electromyography (EMG) can be an additional useful tool for peripheral neuropathy evaluation, although the findings are not specific.

The usefulness of (18) F-FDG in neurosarcoidosis is poor because of the physiologic uptake of (18) F-FDG activity in normal gray matter. However, granulomatous inflammation shows hypermetabolism, whereas neuronal damage presents as hypometabolism. (18) F-FDG-PET may reveal additional occult lesions amenable to biopsy in some patients with inaccessible intracranial lesions, but the literature on (18) F-FDG and neurosarcoidosis is very limited.

2.3.4 Bone sarcoidosis

Bone involvement is a rare manifestation of sarcoidosis usually associated with pulmonary findings. The exact prevalence of bone sarcoidosis is still not known, depending on the studied population and the used diagnostic tools [21]. The prevalence of bone sarcoidosis is between 3% and 5%, above all affecting the phalanges [22].

Both (18)F-FDG-PET/CT and conventional MRI are sensitive in detecting sarcoidosis bone lesions but are not always reliable in differentiating sarcoidosis bone lesions from metastatic disease, thus often requiring bone biopsy [17].

(18) F-FDG-PET/CT is highly sensitive in detecting granulomatous bone marrow infiltration, but an increased (18) F-FDG uptake can mimic metastatic

disease, reducing the specificity of (18) F-FDG-PET/CT when both sarcoidosis and a tumor, which may develop bone metastases, occur in the same patient. Bone assessment in sarcoidosis patients is also performed using MRI, commonly relying on T1-weighted and T2-weighted images. However, routine MRI is not reliable in differentiating sarcoidosis bone lesions from metastatic disease [17].

Multifocal skeletal sarcoidosis may present as a false positive for bone metastases on (18) F-FDG PET/CT since granulomatous bone marrow infiltration may have an uptake of (18) F-FDG, which mimics that of metastatic disease. When false positive findings on (18) F-FDG PET/CT cannot be totally excluded, biopsy or MRI may represent the second choice to achieve diagnosis. Since conventional MRI may not be accurate in distinguishing between sarcoidosis and metastatic bone lesions, it is possible to perform diffusion whole-body MRI: T1-weighted, T2-weighted STIR, and diffusion-weighted imaging (with different *b* values) [17]. The latter is able to evaluate microscopic tissue water motions average at the millimeter scale of MR images. The ADC value reflects the degree of freedom of water movement at the cellular level, which is determined by architectural tissue properties such as cellular density, cellular arrangements, vascularity, extracellular space tissue viscosity, and nuclear/cytoplasmic ratio. Water movement is impeded in many tumors because of their high cellular density and T2 relaxation times, resulting in high signal intensity on diffusion-weighted images and low ADC values [1].

On conventional imaging the pelvic bone lesions appeared with a signal pattern not specific for sarcoidosis bone lesions or metastatic disease (low signal on T1-weighted images and high signal on STIR images). On diffusion-weighted imaging the pelvic bone lesions showed high signal, which is often seen in bone metastases, but the ADC ($<700\ \mu m^2/s$) was too low to be suspicious for metastases from breast cancer [1], which enables to differentiate normal bone marrow from malignant marrow [17, 23, 24].

3. Conclusions

Imaging gives an important contribution to the assessment of prognosis and follow-up in sarcoidosis. FDG-PET/CT is routinely used for the diagnosis, staging, and therapeutic assessment of several malignancies and becomes nowadays a relevant tool for the management of several infectious and inflammatory diseases, such as sarcoidosis. PET can also be a useful tool for the diagnosis of sarcoidosis by identifying potential biopsy sites in organs that might be accessible. FDG-PET/CT plays a crucial role in sarcoidosis disease, especially for the diagnosis of potentially rare extrapulmonary involvement, and is also an interesting tool for assessing therapeutic efficacy of inflammatory diseases and for management of patients.

Conflict of interest

The author declares no conflict of interest.

Thanks

Dedicated to all people who made my dreams come true.

To my beloved parents for the unwavering faith that I would have achieved all the goals I had set for myself.

To those who love me, and loved me, and believed in me, giving me the strength to always go ahead and never give up, standing by my side even when things became difficult.

Often against the wind, but never against my heart.

Author details

Marica Tina Maccarone
AUSL Pescara—Radiology Division, Spirito Santo Hospital Pescara, Italy

*Address all correspondence to: maccaronemarica@hotmail.com

References

[1] Keijsers RG, Veltkamp M, Grutters JC. Chest imaging. Clinics in Chest Medicine. 2015. DOI: 10.1016/j.ccm.2015.08.004

[2] Amin EN, Closser DR, Crouser ED. Current best practice in the management of pulmonary and systemic sarcoidosis. Therapeutic Advances in Respiratory Disease. 2014. DOI: 10.1177/1753465814537367

[3] Mañá J. Molecular imaging in sarcoidosis. Current Opinion in Pulmonary Medicine. 2011. DOI: 10.1097/MCP.0b013e3283480d36

[4] Greco FG, Spagnolo P, Muri M, et al. The value of chest radiograph and computed tomography in pulmonary sarcoidosis. Sarcoidosis, Vasculitis, and Diffuse Lung Diseases. 2014;**31**:108-116

[5] Scadding JG. Prognosis of intrathoracic sarcoidosis in England. A review of 136 cases after five years' observation. British Medical Journal. 1961;**2**:1165-1172. DOI: 10.1136/bmj.2.5261.1165

[6] Basu S, Zhuang H, Torigian DA, Rosenbaum J, Chen W, Alavi A. Functional imaging of inflammatory diseases using nuclear medicine techniques. Seminars in Nuclear Medicine. 2009;**39**(2):124-145. DOI: 10.1053/j.semnuclmed.2008.10.006

[7] Maturu VN, Rayamajhi SJ, Agarwal R, Aggarwal AN, Gupta D, Mittal BR. Role of serial F-18 FDG PET/CT scans in assessing treatment response and predicting relapses in patients with symptomatic sarcoidosis. Sarcoidosis, Vasculitis, and Diffuse Lung Diseases. 2016;**33**(4):372-380

[8] Adams H, Keijsers RG, Korenromp IH, Grutters JC. FDG PET for gauging of sarcoid disease activity. Seminars in Respiratory and Critical Care Medicine. 2014;**35**(3):352-361. DOI: 10.1055/s-0034-1376866

[9] Acar T, Savas R, Kocacelebi K, Ucan ES. Corticosteroid responsive sarcoidosis with multisystemic involvement years after initial diagnosis: A lymphoma mimicker on 18-FDG PET/CT. Journal of Clinical Imaging Science. 2015;**5**:40. DOI: 10.4103/2156-7514.161850

[10] Soussan M, Augier A, Brillet P-Y, Weinmann P, Valeyre D. Functional imaging in extrapulmonary sarcoidosis: FDG-PET/CT and MR features. Clinical Nuclear Medicine. 2013. DOI: 10.1097/RLU.0b013e318279f264

[11] Palestro CJ, Love C. Decreased sensitivity of (18)F-fluorodeoxyglucose imaging in infection and inflammation. Seminars in Nuclear Medicine. 2012;**42**(4):261-266. DOI: 10.1053/j.semnuclmed.2012.04.007

[12] Ramachandraiah V, Aronow W, Chandy D. Pulmonary sarcoidosis: An update. Postgraduate Medicine. 2017;**129**(1):149-158. DOI: 10.1080/00325481.2017.1251818

[13] Aleksonienė R, Zeleckienė I, Matačiūnas M, Puronaitė R, Jurgauskienė L, Malickaitė R, et al. Relationship between radiologic patterns, pulmonary function values and bronchoalveolar lavage fluid cells in newly diagnosed sarcoidosis. Journal of Thoracic Disease. 2017;**9**(1):88-95. DOI: 10.21037/jtd.2017.01.17

[14] Skali H, Schulman AR, Dorbala S. 18F-FDG PET/CT for the assessment of myocardial sarcoidosis. Current Cardiology Reports. 2013

[15] Kataoka S, Momose M, Fukushima K, Serizawa N, Suzuki A, Kondo C, et al. Regional myocardial damage and active inflammation

in patients with cardiac sarcoidosis detected by non-invasive multi-modal imaging. Annals of Nuclear Medicine. 2017;**31**(2):135-143. DOI: 10.1007/s12149-016-1136-1

[16] Zandieh S, Bernt R, Mirzaei S, Haller J, Hergan K. Image fusion between 18F-FDG PET and MRI in cardiac sarcoidosis: A case series. Journal of Nuclear Cardiology. 2016. DOI: 10.1007/s12350-016-0653-6

[17] Vinas FC. Diagnosis and management of neurosarcoidosis. Journal of Clinical Neuroscience. 2001. DOI: 10.1054/jocn.2000.0950

[18] Matsumoto K, Ehara S, Sakaguchi M, Otsuka K, Hasegawa T, Shimada K, et al. Clinical characteristics of late gadolinium enhancement in patients with cardiac sarcoidosis. Osaka City Medical Journal. 2015;**61**(1):9-17

[19] Vargas DL, Stern BJ. Neurosarcoidosis: Diagnosis and management. Seminars in Respiratory and Critical Care Medicine. 2010;**31**(4):419-427. DOI: 10.1055/s-0030-1262210

[20] Tana C, Wegener S, Borys E, Pambuccian S, Tchernev G, Tana M, et al. Challenges in the diagnosis and treatment of neurosarcoidosis. Annals of Medicine. 2015;**47**(7):576-591. DOI: 10.3109/07853890.2015.1093164

[21] Pawate S, Moses H, Sriram S. Presentations and outcomes of neurosarcoidosis: A study of 54 cases. QJM. 2009;**102**(7):449-460. DOI: 10.1093/qjmed/hcp042

[22] Grozdic Milojevic I, Sobic-Saranovic D, Videnovic-Ivanov J, Saranovic D, Odalovic S, Artiko V. FDG PET/CT in bone sarcoidosis. Sarcoidosis, Vasculitis, and Diffuse Lung Diseases. 2016;**33**(1):66-74

[23] Mostard RL, Prompers L, Weijers RE, van Kroonenburgh MJ, Wijnen PA, Geusens PP, et al. F-18 FDG PET/CT for detecting bone and bone marrow involvement in sarcoidosis patients. Clinical Nuclear Medicine. 2012;**37**(1):21-25. DOI: 10.1097/RLU.0b013e3182335f9b

[24] Conte G, Zugni F, Colleoni M, Renne G, Bellomi M, Petralia G. Sarcoidosis with bone involvement mimicking metastatic disease at (18)F-FDG PET/CT: Problem solving by diffusion whole-body MRI. Ecancermedicalscience. 2015;**9**:537. DOI: 10.3332/ecancer.2015.537

Chapter 4

Pathology of Sarcoidosis and Differential Diagnostics of other Granulomatous Diseases

Maria V. Samsonova and Andrey L. Chernyaev

Abstract

Granulomatous diseases are the heterogeneous group of the conditions of different etiologies with a variety of clinic syndromes and morphological features and nonuniform sensitivity to therapy, and the existence of granulomas as general dominate histological expression. Granuloma is indicative of chronic inflammation involving cells of the macrophage system and other inflammatory cells. After the antigen exposure, the activation of T-lymphocytes, macrophages, and epithelioid histiocytes leads to granuloma formation. Granuloma also contains the extracellular matrix produced by fibroblasts, which provide the boundary and isolation of antigen. Their etiology may classify granulomatous diseases as infectious and noninfectious. However, recent studies demonstrate that pathogenic microorganisms may cause the granuloma formation in diseases previously considered as noninfectious. In some cases, differentiation between infectious and noninfectious processes may be problematic. This chapter aims to highlight the multiformity of granulomatous diseases, characterize the pathologic features of different infectious and noninfectious granulomatosis, and delineate the diagnostic approach.

Keywords: lung pathology, granulomatous diseases, sarcoidosis, infection, vasculitis

1. Introduction

Granulomatous diseases are a heterogeneous group of the conditions of various etiologies with a variety of clinic syndromes and morphological features, nonuniform sensitivity to therapy, and the existence of granulomas. Granuloma is indicative of chronic inflammation involving cells of the macrophage system and other inflammatory cells. After antigen exposure, the activation of T-lymphocytes, macrophages, and epithelioid histiocytes lead to granuloma formation. Granulomas also contain the extracellular matrix produced by fibroblasts, which provide the boundary and isolation of antigens. Their etiology may classify granulomatous diseases as infectious and noninfectious. However, recent studies demonstrate that pathogenic microorganisms may cause the granuloma formation in diseases previously considered as noninfectious. In some cases, differentiation between infectious and noninfectious processes may be problematic. This chapter aims to highlight the multiple forms of granulomatous diseases, characterize the pathologic features of different infectious and noninfectious granulomatosis, and delineate the diagnostic approach.

IntechOpen

The term granuloma comes from the Latin word "*granulum*" which means "grain," and the Greek suffix ""*-oma*" used to refer to its nodular formation. Granuloma is a nodular defined formation. This term designates compact cell aggregates on microscopy; granulomas may consist of histiocytes and/or epithelioid cells, giant multinucleated cells, and other inflammatory cells (lymphocytes, neutrophils, and eosinophils). Epithelioid and giant multinucleated cells are monocytes/macrophages derivatives; the former represents good differentiated secretory cells, while the latter specializes in phagocytosis [1]. Giant multinucleated cells are formed by fusion or incomplete cell division, proven in experimental studies [2]; moreover, foreign-body giant cells are formed earlier, than Langhans cells. Lymphocytes are located mainly at the periphery of a granuloma and are represented by T-cells while B-lymphocytes are scattered outside the granuloma. Depending on the disease, T-lymphocytes are predominantly represented by T-helpers 1 and 2 or cytotoxic T-suppressors.

Granulomatous diseases are the heterogeneous group of the diseases of different etiology with a variety of clinic syndromes and morphological features, nonuniform sensitivity to therapy [3]. This chapter aims to highlight the variety of granulomatous lung diseases, to characterize the key morphological features of various diseases of infectious and noninfectious nature, as well as to delineate the diagnostic approach. First, the granulomatous diseases, with arising granulomas which do not lead to necrosis development, with some exceptions are mentioned.

2. Sarcoidosis

Lung lesions in sarcoidosis are described in 90% of cases. The morphological feature of sarcoidosis is epithelioid cell granuloma, which is a compact formation of mononuclear phagocytes (macrophages and epithelioid cells). Each sarcoid granuloma has certain stages of development. These stages are as follows:

1. Early or macrophage granuloma, sometimes with a few histiocytes, lymphocytes, or neutrophils (**Figure 1**);

2. Granuloma with an epithelioid cell cluster in the center and macrophages at the periphery;

3. Lymphocytic epithelioid granuloma;

4. The appearance of giant multinucleated cells (at first foreign-body giant cells, followed by Langhans cells);

5. Early cell necrosis in the center of the granuloma due to nuclear pycnosis, the formation of apoptotic bodies, and epithelial cell necrosis;

6. Central fibrinoid, granular, coagulative ischemic necrosis, as a rule, in small foci;

7. Granuloma with fibrosis (or hyalinosis); silver stain is used to detect reticulin fibers;

8. Hyalinized granuloma.

The process of granuloma organization begins at the periphery; that is why they have well-defined, "stamped" appearance (**Figure 2**).

Moreover, in sarcoidosis, granulomas of different "age" may be frequently found in the same samples; granulomas often form conglomerates (**Figure 3**) [4].

A significant number of lymphocytes in lung tissue in patients with sarcoidosis are predominantly represented by T-cells. It is useful to evaluate the bronchioloalveolar lavage (BAL) while carrying out the differential diagnosis: In sarcoidosis

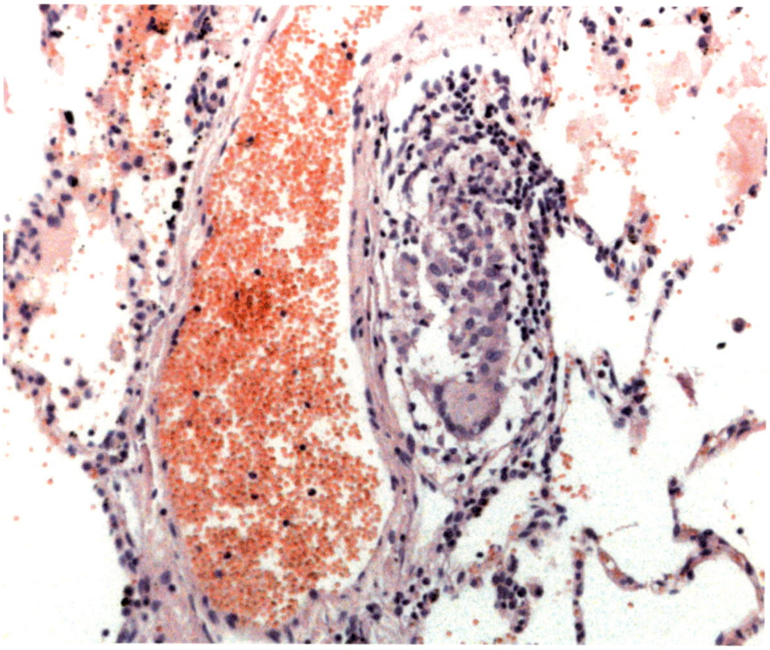

Figure 1.
Macrophage granuloma.

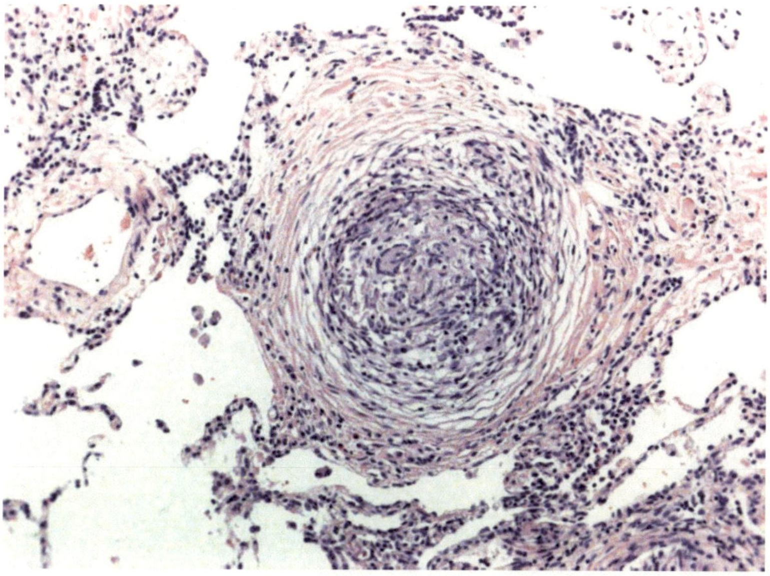

Figure 2.
Typical "stamped" sarcoid granuloma. H&E.

T-helpers predominate. Giant cells in granulomas may contain cytoplasmic inclusions, such as asteroid bodies, Schaumann bodies, or crystalloid structures. These inclusions are characteristic of sarcoidosis, but they are not pathognomonic, as they may be found in other granulomatous diseases [5]. The end stage of sarcoidosis is characterized with prominent fibrosis, sometimes with honeycombing, in which only the remnants of granulomas could be found (**Figure 4**).

Typical locations of granulomas in sarcoidosis are perilymphatic or subpleural zones. Granulomas in bronchi and bronchioles may be found in 15–55% cases of sarcoidosis. Furthermore, granulomas are often located in the vessel wall; the frequency of granulomatous vasculitis may reach 69% (**Figure 5**). In these cases,

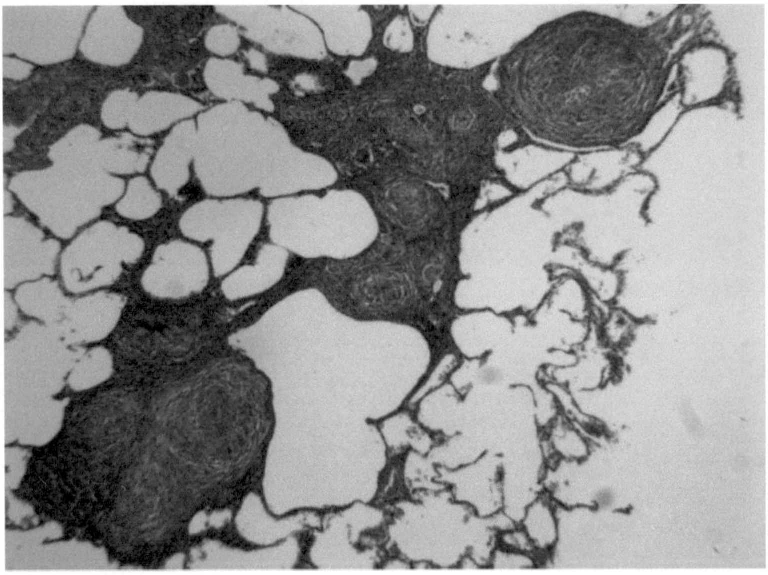

Figure 3.
Multiple well-defined epithelioid cell sarcoid granulomas, forming the conglomerates. H&E.

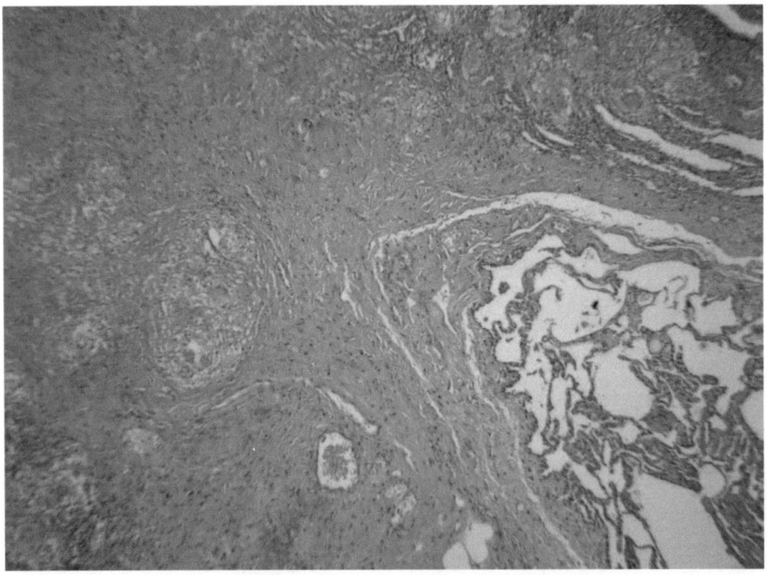

Figure 4.
Late-stage sarcoidosis with prominent fibrosis and remnants of granulomas. H&E.

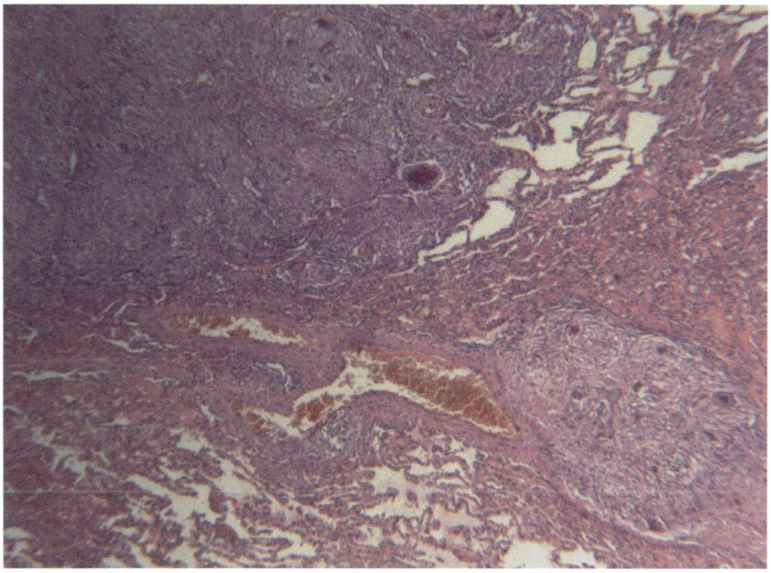

Figure 5.
Granulomatous vasculitis in sarcoidosis. H&E.

sarcoidosis should be differentiated from necrotizing sarcoid granulomatosis. The latter is attributed by some authors to the nodular form of sarcoidosis; necrosis is typical for this disease [6].

Summing up, sarcoidosis is characterized by sharply defined, "stamped" granulomas located along the lymphatic vessels with concentric fibrosis around the granulomas and hyalinosis inside and between the granulomas, also by granulomatous vasculitis, the absence of chronic interstitial inflammation outside the granulomatous lesions, and the absence of organized pneumonia foci. Apart from sarcoidosis, a so-called nonspecific sarcoid reaction occurs in the form of epithelioid cell granulomatosis. It is usually observed in regional lymph nodes, but may also be found in lung tissue in pseudotumors, malignant neoplasms, parasitic diseases, and tuberculosis. Histologically, the sarcoid reaction is characterized by its locality and a topical relationship with these pathological processes.

2.1 Hypersensitivity pneumonitis

The pathogenesis of hypersensitivity pneumonitis is based on type III (immunocomplex) and type IV immunological reactions in the lung during allergen inhalation. The etiological factor of this medical condition is usually thermophilic bacteria, fungi, and animal proteins. Other bacteria and their products, amoeba, and some chemicals are much less likely to cause the disease. In case of hypersensitivity pneumonitis, granulomas are poorly formed, and loose, composed of histiocytes, lymphocytes and, multinucleated cells; some eosinophils may also be identified (**Figure 6**) [7].

Unlike sarcoidosis, peribronchiolar localization of granulomas is typical for hypersensitivity pneumonitis. The triad of pathomorphological features characterizes hypersensitivity pneumonitis: Nonspecific interstitial pneumonia in the peribronchiolar zones, non-necrotizing histiocytic (giant cell) granulomas, and foci of bronchiolitis obliterans. "Needle-like" inclusions are often observed inside giant cells in the granuloma areas and the alveoli in hypersensitivity pneumonitis. In the late, fibrous stage of the disease, the histological features are similar to those in

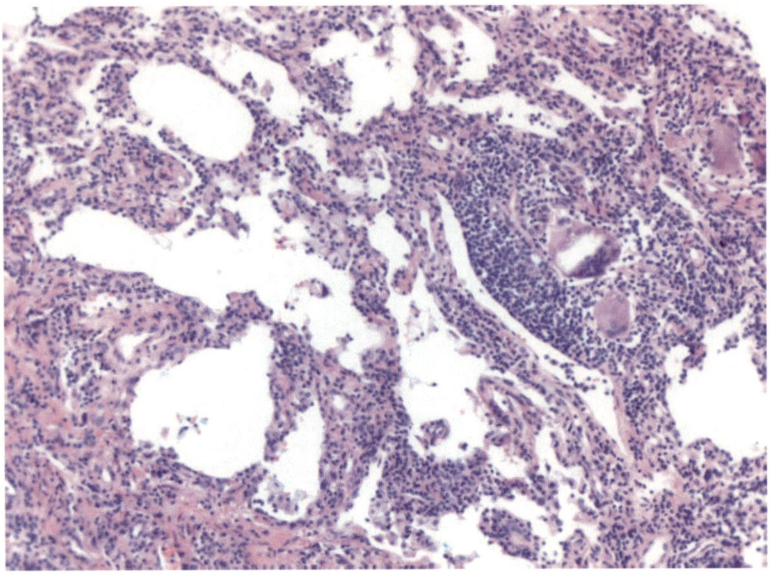

Figure 6.
Hypersensitivity pneumonitis: Ill-defined granuloma consisting of giant multinucleated cells with needle-like structures surrounded by lymphocytes, lymphocytic infiltration of interalveolar septa. H&E.

usual interstitial pneumonia, only scattered giant cells or remnants of granulomas may be found in the fibrotic areas or in the honeycomb zones in hypersensitivity pneumonitis [8].

2.2 Chronic allergic disease caused by metals

Chronic berylliosis is an allergic granulomatosis. Granulomas are similar to those in sarcoidosis and may be slightly larger. As in sarcoidosis, granulomas have perilymphatic location, and lymph nodes are usually affected. The same variant of granulomatosis may develop as a result of zirconium exposure. The diagnosis should be based on the clinical history and lymphocyte transformation test [9].

2.3 Polyangiit with granulomatosis

In our opinion, of particular difficulty is **the differential diagnosis of necrotizing granulomatosis**. Infectious disease, as one of the most common causes of necrotizing granulomatosis, should be differentiated from polyangiitis with granulomatosis (previously Wegener's granulomatosis), aspiration pneumonia, and less often from nodular form of rheumatoid arthritis, necrotizing sarcoid granulomatosis (NSG), lung infarction, and lymphomatoid granulomatosis [10]. Despite the specific histological changes in these diseases, there is, however, an overlap, and only a combination of histological features help in the final diagnosis. **Infectious necrotizing granuloma** usually has smooth contours, commonly eosinophilic necrosis, surrounded by a rim of histiocytes and giant multinucleated cells. By contrast, in polyangiitis with granulomatosis, the necrosis zone has uneven contours resembling a geographical map, with a large amount of cellular debris, which gives the necrosis a "dirty" appearance (**Figure 7**).

Necrotic areas are also surrounded by a histiocytic rim; however, giant cells are usually few in number and are scattered without forming compact granulomas. A characteristic feature of polyangiitis with granulomatosis is the necrotizing vasculitis with fibrinoid necrosis of the media (**Figure 8**);

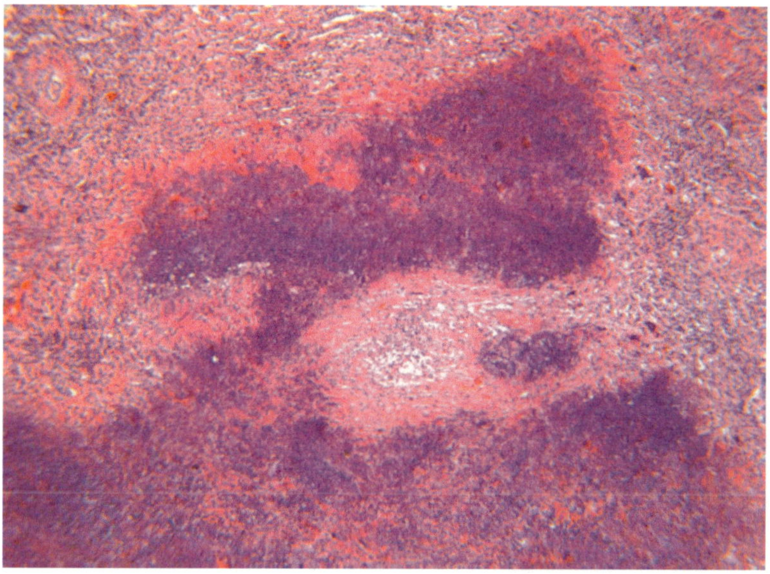

Figure 7.
Polyangiit with granulomatosis: "geographic" necrosis with cell debris. H&E.

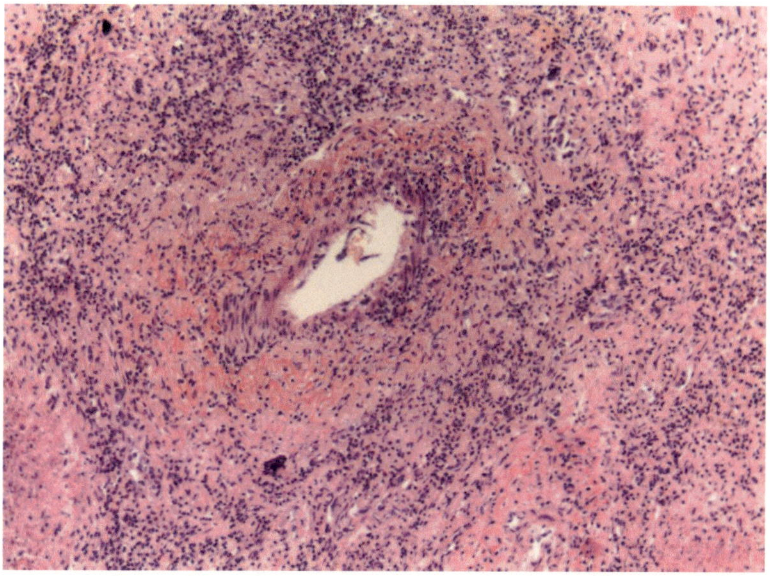

Figure 8.
Polyangiit with granulomatosis: Fibrinoid necrosis of the vessel wall with lymphocytic infiltration. H&E.

Such vessels are observed in the inflammation; the damage to the vessel wall is often eccentric; also, the branches of the pulmonary arteries and veins are affected in this disease. The capillaritis, accompanied by intra-alveolar hemorrhages, may also be observed. Necrotizing vasculitis may often be found in the inflammation and necrosis, but this is also in the infectious granulomatosis; therefore, to confirm the diagnosis of polyangiitis with granulomatosis, it is necessary to carefully evaluate the vessels outside necrosis, and additional stains are recommended to identify elastic tissue (Verhoeff-van Gieson stain and others). In contrast to infectious granulomatosis, lymph node involvement is not typical for polyangiitis with granulomatosis [11].

2.4 Allergic angiitis with granulomatosis

Necrotizing granulomatosis is also seen in (previously, Churg-Strauss syndrome), in combination with necrotizing vasculitis and eosinophilic pneumonia. Granulomas in allergic angiitis with granulomatosis are well formed; with central necrosis containing many eosinophils, there is also eosinophilic infiltration of the blood vessel walls and bronchioles, necrotizing vasculitis with eosinophils, and giant multinucleated cells present. However, additional clinical and laboratory data are necessary to determine the diagnosis, because the classical triad (granulomatosis, necrotizing vasculitis, and eosinophilic pneumonia) is rarely found in lungs.

2.5 Rheumatoid arthritis

Furthermore, necrotizing pulmonary granulomas may form in rheumatoid arthritis; however, the diagnosis in this case should be made with caution. First of all, one should take into account clinical data, since nodular forms of rheumatoid arthritis develop only in the active phase in seropositive patients with severe articular syndrome. As a rule, necrosis is eosinophilic, cell debris is usually located between the necrosis and the surrounding rim of histiocytes; it may be combined with vasculitis, but necrotizing vasculitis is not characteristic for this disease (**Figure 9**) [12]. The described histological features are practically indistinguishable from infectious granulomatosis; moreover, rare clinical cases of rheumatoid arthritis and tuberculosis combination have been described, and therefore, the infection must be thoroughly excluded.

2.6 Necrotizing sarcoid granulomatosis (NSG)

Infectious granulomatosis should also be differentiated from NSG. Some characteristics of the latter are likened to those seen in polyangiitis with granulomatosis. NSG is characterized by the interstitial necrosis, which is often eosinophilic, but

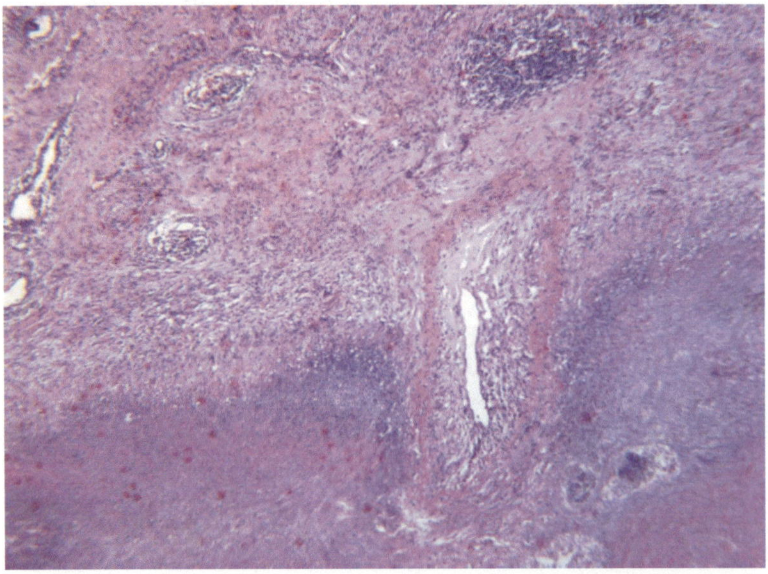

Figure 9.
Rheumatoid arthritis: Extensive necrosis with rims of histiocytes at the periphery and lymphoid infiltration of vessel wall. H&E.

sometimes may contain cellular debris. However, necrosis in NSG is combined with the non-necrotizing sarcoid-type granulomas, consisting mainly of epithelioid and giant multinucleated cells with just a small number of lymphocytes. These granulomas tend to merge and are often located near blood vessels or in its walls, but not causing vasculitis (**Figure 10**) [6]. The following symptom triad is obligatory for the NSG diagnosis: sarcoid-type granulomas, granulomatous vasculitis, and necrotizing inflammation.

Since necrosis in infectious granulomatosis may be of a coagulation type, pulmonary infarction should also be a part of the differential diagnosis. In the stage of organization, infarction may be surrounded by fibroblasts and inflammatory cells, resembling granulomatous inflammation. As a rule, in lung resection specimens with pulmonary infarction, thrombi can be detected in the branches of the pulmonary artery that caused the development of a pulmonary infarction [13].

2.7 Granulomatous inflammation caused by infectious agents

2.7.1 Fungi

Fungi that cause deep mycoses, as a rule, do not form granulomas in the lungs. In most cases, fungi such as *Aspergillus, Candida*, and some others cause local mycetoma, diffuse invasive mycosis, or allergic reactions (allergic bronchopulmonary aspergillosis/mycosis). The granulomatous response in these fungi infections is rare [14].

2.7.1.1 Histoplasmosis

Histoplasmosis is caused by *H. capsulatum* (North America, river valleys) and *H. duboisii* (Africa), which are budding yeast cells with a diameter of 2–4 μm. Microorganisms are found in the cytoplasm of macrophages, histiocytes, and necrotic debris. Its capsule is stained with Giemsa or PAS reaction. Both organisms

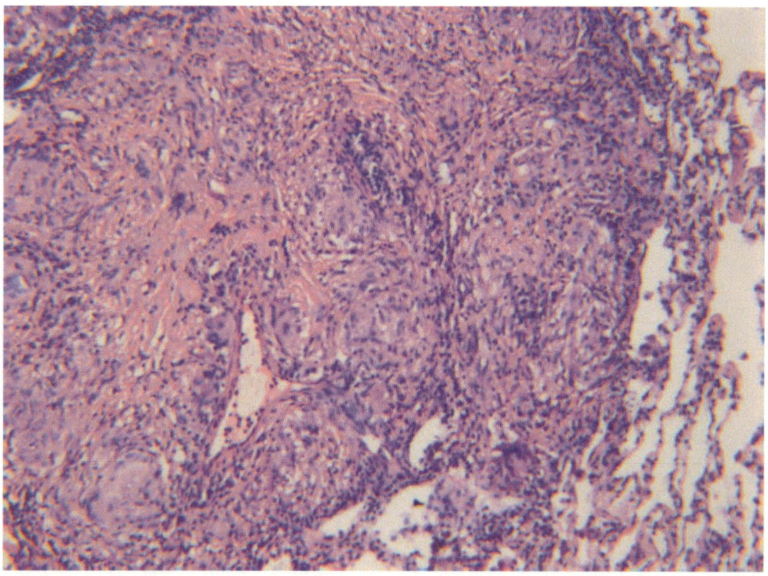

Figure 10.
Necrotizing sarcoid granulomatosis: Granulomatous vasculitis. H&E.

cause the formation of epithelioid cell granulomas; however, necrotizing granulomatosis is more often described in *H. capsulatum* infection [15].

2.7.1.2 Cryptococcosis (European blastomycosis)

Cryptococcus neoformans is ubiquitous; it is found in soil and pigeon excrements. The fungal cell is of 4–7 μm in size, replicates by budding, and is stained with H&E, mucicarmin, and PAS. Cryptococci cause a spectrum of various changes in the lungs. A typical granulomatous reaction presents with confluent non-necrotizing granulomas, many multinucleated giant cells, and a mild inflammatory reaction; giant cells are located mainly outside the granulomas and contain cryptococcal cells (**Figure 11**).

These fungi can also be located inside necrotizing granulomas (cryptococcomas) resembling those with mycobacterial and other types of fungal infections (**Figure 12**). In immunocompromised individuals, cryptococcal cells are found inside the alveoli, in their walls, and in the interstitium, without marked inflammatory reaction; some scattered multinucleated giant cells can be found [9].

2.7.1.3 Coccidiosis

Coccidia most often lead to necrotizing granuloma formation; the eosinophilic reaction may be marked or absent; numerous neutrophils may be observed. Like in other infections, granulomas are located peribronchiolar or with destroyed bronchioles. This process is accompanied by the formation of small non-necrotizing granulomas at the periphery. *Coccidia* are usually found in the center of necrotizing granulomas, they consist of large spherical structures (spherules) containing yeast-like structures (endospores). Endospores of various sizes can be located in necrosis or cellular debris, resembling other fungal infections. The detection of spherules and endospores favor the diagnosis of coccidiosis. Like *Histoplasma*, *Coccidia* do not grow in vitro; thus, the diagnosis can only be made by histological examination [15].

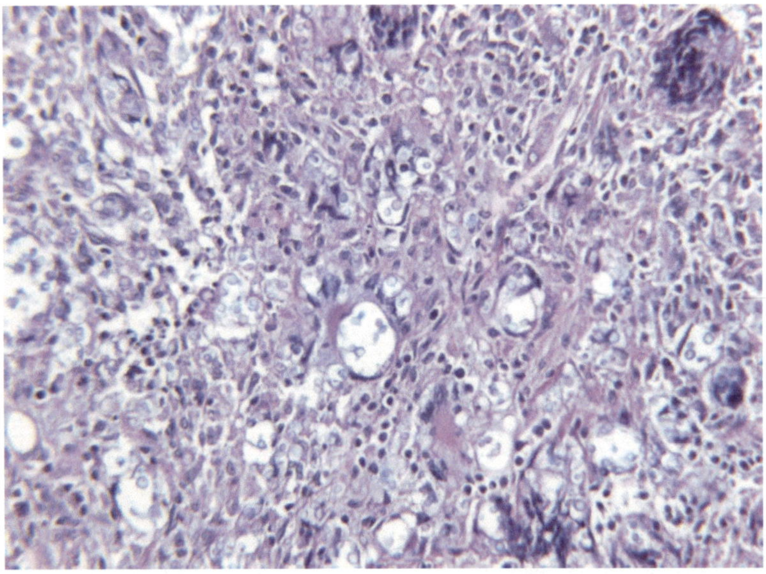

Figure 11.
Cryptococci cells and multinucleated giant cells in a granuloma. Combined stain of alcian blue and PAS.

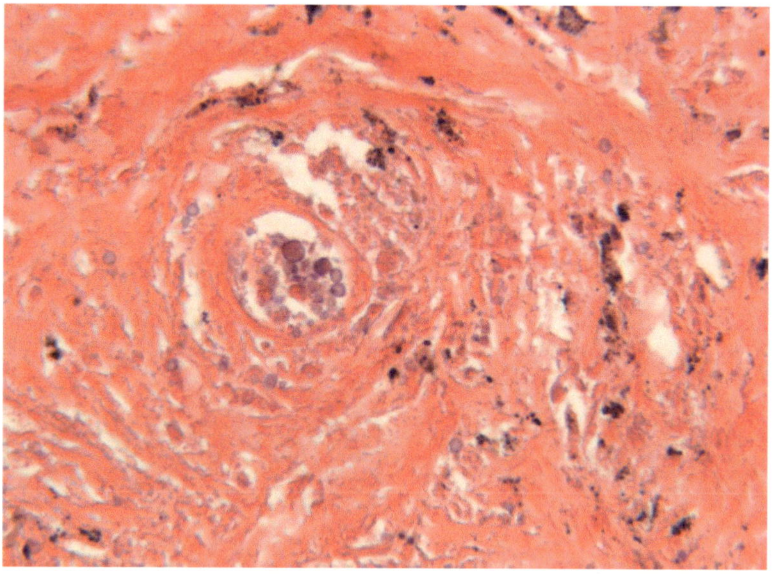

Figure 12.
Necrotizing granuloma fragment with cryptococci cells. H&E.

2.7.1.4 Blastomycosis

Blastomycosis is a rare disease, and this diagnosis may be suspected when granulomatosis or giant cell lesion in combination with severe acute inflammation is detected. Blastomycosis is characterized by basophilic necrosis rich in cellular debris in contrast to eosinophilic or slightly "dirty" infectious necrotizing granulomas. Blastomycosis is often a bronchiolocentric process. Large, thick-walled, yeast-like *Blastomyces* cells can be detected in H&E and also mucicarmin staining. Active budding is a distinctive feature of the microorganism; nuclear material (multiple nucleoli) can also be found inside the cells, but these signs are not always observed. In this regard, compared to *Histoplasma* and *Cryptococci* cells and *coccidial* endospores, *Blastomyces* cells are larger but still smaller than *coccidial* spherules [15].

2.7.1.5 Pneumocystosis

Most pathologists are familiar with the conventional picture of pneumonia caused by *Pneumocystis*, but 5–17% describe the formation of an ill-defined intraalveolar epithelioid or histiocytic granuloma around the eosinophilic exudate, sometimes without exudate; the formation of well-defined granulomas with central necrosis or without it is also possible [16, 17]. Sometimes the granulomatous reaction in pneumocystis pneumonia is a foreign-body granulomatosis (**Figure 13**).

2.8 Parasites

Dirofilaria is one of the most common parasites that lead to the granulomatous inflammation in lungs. This nematode infects dogs more commonly, but the disease can also occur in humans, as the infection is transmitted through an insect bite; the larva enters the right heart and into the pulmonary arteries during embolism, causing thrombosis of the latter with an infarct-like necrosis development (**Figure 14**). In one-third of the cases, granulomas are formed in the adjacent lung

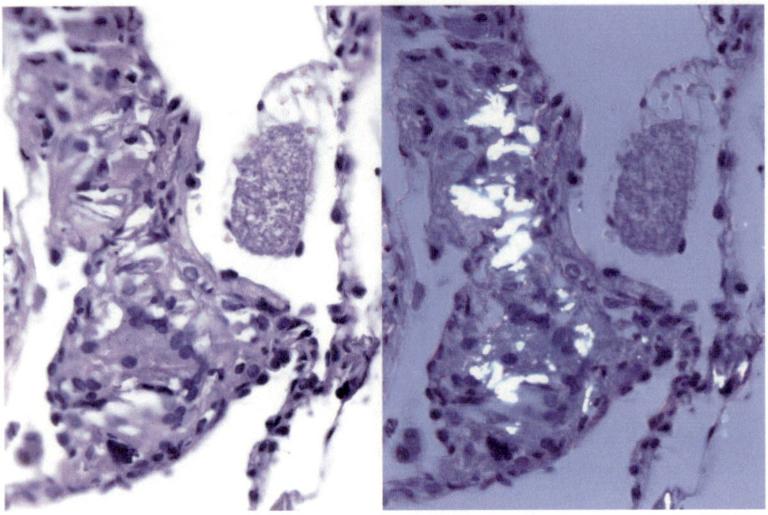

Figure 13.
Perivascular foreign-body granuloma (talcosis) in a case of pneucystic pneumonia in a drug abuser. H&E in bright field versus polarization.

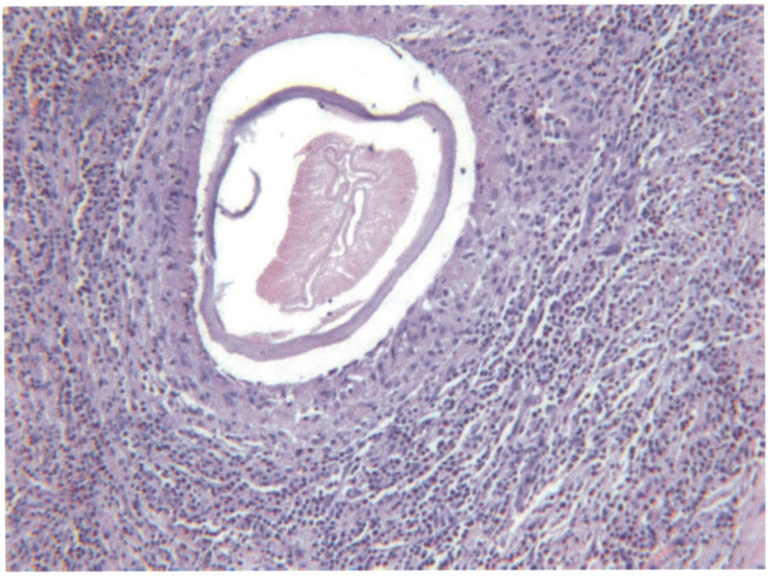

Figure 14.
Dirofilaria *larva in the pulmonary artery, infiltration of plasma cells and eosinophils. H&E.*

tissue, necrotizing or non-necrotizing vasculitis is observed in half of the cases, and two-thirds of the cases demonstrate eosinophilic infiltration [18].

2.9 Tuberculosis

Tuberculosis is caused by members of the *Mycobacterium tuberculosis* family, namely, *M. tuberculosis, M. bovis,* and *M. africanum*, which belong to the group of rapidly growing mycobacteria. The virulence of these microorganisms varies from moderate to highly virulent strains. Changes observed in the lungs in tuberculosis patients can be very diverse ranging from common necrotizing granulomas, miliary necrotizing granulomas to non-necrotizing granulomas, tuberculoma, and healed

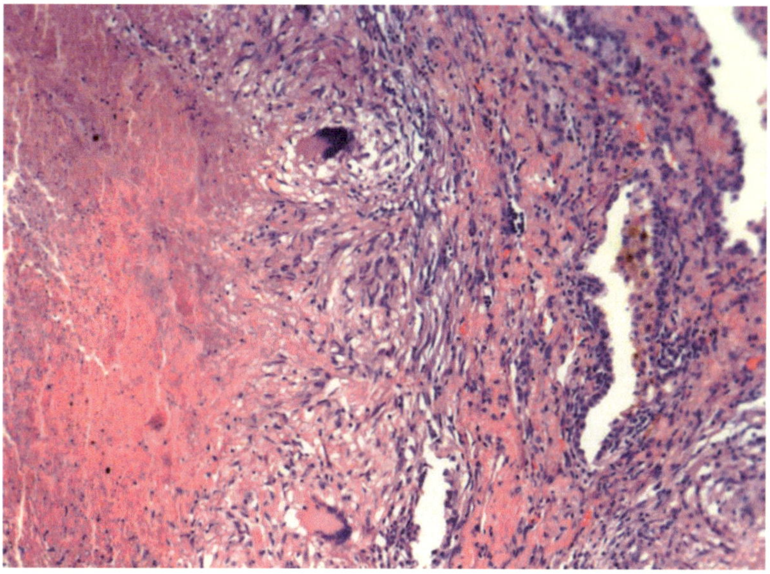

Figure 15.
Tuberculous necrotizing granuloma with lymphocytes, histiocytes, and giant multinucleated Langhans at the periphery. H&E.

fibrosus granulomas, all of these depend on the virulence on the one hand and the immune defense status on the other (**Figure 15**) [19]. Granulomas in tuberculosis usually have a bronchiolocentric localization, but it should be kept in mind that this could be the case in any infectious granulomatosis and even in sarcoidosis. Histological features in tuberculosis are indistinguishable from those in non-tuberculous granulomatosis. This was confirmed in a study by Corpe and Stergus, in which 27 pathologists, specializing in the mycobacterial disease diagnostics, were asked to evaluate 25 histological slides without information about culture-confirmed infection. In most cases, it was not possible to distinguish between tuberculosis and mycobacteriosis [20]. Thus, the tuberculosis diagnosis **should be based** on the identification and subsequent determination of the type of *Mycobacterium*.

2.10 Non-tuberculosis mycobacteriosis

Non-tuberculosis mycobacteriosis is an inflammation caused by mycobacteria not belonging to the *Mycobacterium tuberculosis* family; those are *M. avium, M. fortuitum, M. gordonae, M. kansasii, M. xenopi*, and *M. marinum*, also designated as MAC complex. Unlike *Mycobacterium tuberculosis*, these mycobacteria can be detected intracellularly in macrophages (histiocytes), and they can be numerous in immunocompromised individuals. The diagnosis is made based on acid-fast stain, cultural or molecular biological tests. As mentioned above, the histological changes are often similar to those in tuberculosis. Non-necrotizing granulomas, histiocytic granulomas, and granulomas consisting of foamy and granular macrophages containing mycobacteria can also be detected. Solovieva et al. have described the following spectrum of histological changes in mycobacteriosis:

- tuberculous granuloma—epithelioid cell tissue, variable number of Langhans cells and the necrosis intensity, few mycobacteria;

- a reactive, necrotizing multibacillarity—weak inflammatory response, abundance of mycobacteria in the necrosis area;

- multibacillary histiocytosis—diffuse macrophage infiltration with an intracellular abundance of mycobacteria, no necrosis;
- multibacillary minimal histiocytosis—a mild inflammatory reaction with an intracellular abundance of mycobacteria;
- histoid lesion—nodular clusters of spindle-shaped macrophages with an abundance of mycobacteria;
- nonspecific granulation tissue;
- acute purulent abscess [21].

The MAC-hypersensitivity-like disease has also been described (or "hot tub lung"); it is caused by mycobacteria of the MAC complex, and associated with the use of sauna and showers, which leads to the aerosol inhalation. The histological features of this disease are similar to the hypersensitivity pneumonitis changes [22].

2.11 Differential diagnostics of granulomatous lung diseases

A variety of diseases leading to granulomatosis determine certain difficulties in conducting the differential diagnostics even when resectional (surgical, video-assisted) biopsies are performed, which allows obtaining a sufficient amount of material for histological evaluation [23]. However, it is not always possible to establish the cause of granulomatous inflammation. According to Ulbright and Katzenstein, who analyzed 86 solitary lung granulomas detected by X-ray, the infection caused by acid-resistant mycobacteria or fungi was confirmed in 70%. In 25 cases, the infectious etiology was not proven, while two patients were diagnosed with hyalinized granuloma, one patient—with polyangiitis with granulomatosis, and in 22 cases, it was not possible to classify the process. Also, a significant similarity of histological changes in infectious granulomas and polyangiitis with granulomatosis was found; it may be possible that the latter was a reflection of the immune response disorders to an infectious agent which could no longer be found in the tissue samples. This means that polyangiitis with granulomatosis and other lung angiitis diagnoses should be made with extreme caution in cases with solitary nodes while no damage to other organs is detected. In such cases, a thorough examination of patients and follow-up should be recommended [24].

Mukhopadhyay et al. conducted a multicenter retrospective study of 500 biopsies from 10 clinics in the United States, Britain, Austria, Brazil, Japan, Turkey, and India with pulmonary granulomatosis. During the biopsy analysis, a specific diagnosis was established in 58% of the cases: most commonly sarcoidosis (27%) and mycobacterial infection (25%) were detected. Mycobacterial infection was proved in 18% outside the USA versus 8% in the USA; on the contrary, fungal infection amounted to 19% in the USA (most often histoplasmosis) versus 4% in other countries. Fungi were commonly detected by histological examination, while mycobacterial infection was confirmed in culture. In 42% of the cases, the etiological factor of granulomatosis was not established.

This study, in our opinion, is extremely interesting: First of all, it indicates the predominance of sarcoidosis and infectious granulomatous inflammation in the structure of granulomatous diseases according to histological analysis conducted in different countries and geographical regions. Fungal infection more often caused granulomatous inflammation in the United States, while mycobacterial infection was more often diagnosed in other countries, which is a reflection of the infection endemicity. It is crucial to send the specimen simultaneously to the histological and microbiological laboratory in all cases when a granulomatous disease is suspected, that will definitely improve the quality of the etiological diagnosis. According to this study, the cause of granulomatosis was not established in more than a third of clinical cases even after histological examination [22].

The frequency of infectious granulomatosis is high. When all other causes based on the clinical history, clinical syndromes, laboratory tests, and specific morphological features mentioned above are excluded, the remaining granulomatous diseases are most likely to be attributed to infectious.

An important issue in the differential diagnosis of the infectious granulomatosis diseases is the detection of an infectious agent in microscopical slides. To achieve this, it is necessary and obligatory to perform additional stains. One can detect fungal infection, first of all, by carefully evaluating hematoxylin- and eosin-stained (H&E) slides. Most fungi, such as *Cryptococcus*, *Blastomyces*, *Cocidioides*, and *Aspergillus*, can be found in H&E slides, more often in necrosis areas than in the adjacent lung tissue. The pathologist should select slides with necrosis present when ordering additional stains. Grocott's methenamine silver stain and the PAS reaction are the most commonly used for the fungal infection diagnosis confirmation, also alcian blue (Mouri), the basic brown stains (Shubich's method), or the combined stain of PAS with alcian blue [14].

Ziehl-Neelsen stain is used to diagnose mycobacterial infection; however, mycobacteria are usually few in number, and their search is quite time-consuming. Alternative stains with auramine or auramine/rhodamine increase the sensitivity of the method, but these techniques require fluorescence microscopy (**Figure 16a** and **b**). To increase the detection of mycobacteria, Ulbright and Katzenstein recommend performing staining in at least two blocks [24]. Gomori silver or Warthin-Starry stains are recommended for syphilis diagnosis [9].

One of the open questions is whether there are additional opportunities, modern techniques for diagnosing infectious granulomatosis. Immunohistochemistry is available, but it has several limitations, namely cross-reactivity, as well as the antibody accessibility, especially for rare microorganisms. *In situ* hybridization may

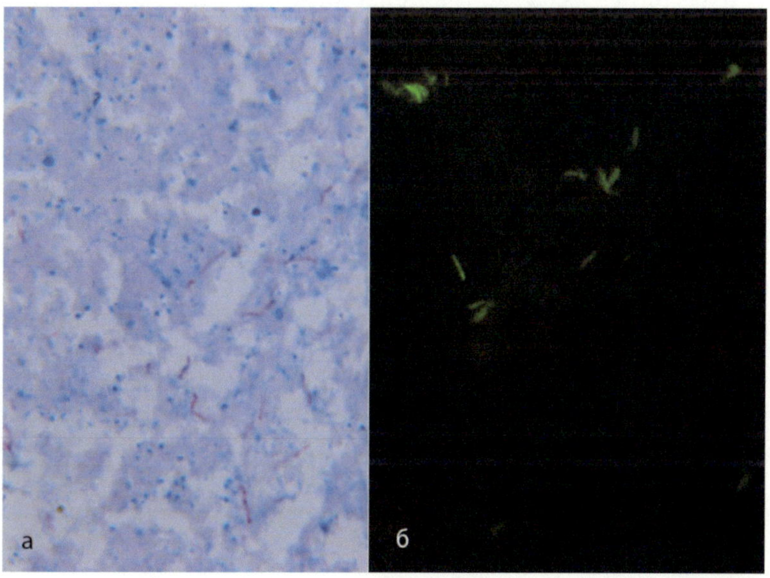

Figure 16.
Acid-fast mycobacteria: (a) Ziehl-Neelsen stain and (b) auramine/rhodamine (fluorescence).

also be useful, but not for the detection, but for the identification of fungi found in traditionally stained slides. Real-time PCR can be performed on paraffin sections for tuberculosis diagnostics; the specificity of this method is 99%; however, the sensitivity amounts to only 65%. Nevertheless, when the same method is used to detect mycobacteria tuberculosis in the cerebrospinal fluid, urine, or bronchoalveolar lavage, the sensitivity is more than 90%. Thus, this technique is useful and confirms the diagnosis if mycobacteria are detected, but PCR does not exclude the tuberculosis diagnosis if the result is negative. In addition, it does not allow detecting non-tuberculous mycobacteria. According to Aubry, the cultural study remains the "gold standard" for non-tuberculous mycobacteriosis diagnostics, and, according to their research, indicates that in more than 75% of cases, the only method to confirm mycobacteriosis was in culture [10].

The etiological factor remains unclear in 30–40% of infectious granulomatosis even in leading US university clinics despite a complete histological evaluation of lung tissue slides, as well as correlations with clinical, microbiological, and serological data. In this regard, the question of diagnostic significance of these diseases arises. Ulbright and Katzenstein propose that such cases represent infectious granulomas in which the microorganism was destroyed and/or removed by means of the developed inflammatory process [24]. A retrospective analysis of necrotizing granulomas showed that patients who did not receive further specific therapy were still alive and did not demonstrate any clinical symptoms. The same hypothesis is confirmed by Aubry who notes that even if new foci appear in these patients, poor outcomes were not detected [10]. It can be recommended to pathologists to give a descriptive histological conclusion indicating the presence/absence of necrosis, the absence of detected microorganisms: "The disease etiology is most likely to be infectious, special stains for the microorganism detection are negative."

When a granulomatous disease is suspected and lung resection is performed, it is necessary to save some specimen tissue unfixed for possible cultural study, and use the quick freeze method at -70°C for subsequent DNA and RNA analyses, if available. In the differential diagnosis of granulomatous diseases, first of all, one should determine whether the granuloma is infectious, or there are signs of other diseases, including Wegener's granulomatosis. If a specific diagnosis is excluded, it is crucial to perform special stains for microorganism detection, it is preferable to stain sections from at least two blocks, while making sure that necrosis foci are present in the material. If the microorganism detection is not possible at the first glance, we recommend evaluating the slides again at a higher magnification, and also using an additional block for staining. When negative result is received, but clinical data are in favor of tuberculosis or other infections, PCR is suggested. Additional cultural and serological studies, which would be able to exclude the infectious process, should be performed in case of another negative result obtained. Nevertheless, according to this algorithm results, a certain part of granulomatous diseases appears to have an uncertain etiology.

In conclusion, we would like to emphasize that the differential diagnosis of granulomatous pulmonary diseases is not so easy for pathologists. To exclude or prove the infectious disease, the pathologist should carefully examinate special stained specimens. Noninfectious granulomatous lung disease should be proved, taking into consideration both clinical and radiological data. Finally, from the pathologic point of view, there are the situations for which a specific diagnosis cannot be made. Multidisciplinary approach sometimes is recommended for decision-making.

Author details

Maria V. Samsonova[1*] and Andrey L. Chernyaev[2]

1 Department of Pathology of Federal State Budgetary Institution, Pulmonology Scientific Research Institute under Federal Medical and Biological Agency of Russian Federation, Moscow, Russia

2 Division of Fundamental Pulmonology of Federal State Budgetary Institution, Pulmonology Scientific Research Institute under Federal Medical and Biological Agency of Russian Federation, Moscow, Russia

*Address all correspondence to: samary@mail.ru

References

[1] Muller H, Kruger S. Immunohistochemical analysis of cell composition and in situ cytokine expression in HIV- and non-HIV-associated tuberculosis lymphadenitis. Immunobiology. 1994;**191**:354-368. DOI: 10.1016/s0171-2985(11)80441-9

[2] Enelow RI, Sullivan GW, Carper HT, Mandell GL. Induction of multinucleated giant cell formation from in vitro culture of human monocytes with interleukin-3 and interferon-gamma: Comparison with other stimulating factors. American Journal of Respiratory Cell and Molecular Biology. 1992;**6**:57-62. DOI: 10.1165/ajrcmb/6.1.57

[3] Strukov AI, OYA K. Granulomatous Inflammation and Granulomatous Diseases. Moscow. Medizina: AMS USSR; 1989. p. 184

[4] Hunninghake GW, Costabel U, Ando M, et al. Statement on sarcoidosis. Joint Statement of the American Thoracic Society (ATS), the European Respiratory Society (ERS) and the World Association of Sarcoidosis and Other Granulomatous Disorders (WASOG) adopted by the ATS Board of Directors and by the ERS Executive Committee, February 1999. American Journal of Respiratory and Critical Care Medicine. 1999;**160**:736-755. DOI: 10.1164/ajrccm.160.2.ats4-99

[5] Gal AA, Koss MN. The pathology of sarcoidosis. Current Opinion in Pulmonary Medicine. 2002;**8**(5):445-451. DOI: 10.1097/00063198-200209000-00018

[6] Popper HH, Klemen H, Colby TV, Churg A. Necrotizing sarcoid granulomatosis – is it different from nodular sarcoidosis? Pneumologie. 2003;**57**(5):268-271. DOI: 10.1055/s-2003-39365

[7] Coleman A, Colby TV. Histologic diagnosis of extrinsic allergic alveolitis. The American Journal of Surgical Pathology. 1988;**12**(7):514-518. DOI: 10.1097/00000478-198807000-00002

[8] Barrios RJ. Hypersensitivity pneumonitis: Histopathology. Archives of Pathology & Laboratory Medicine. 2008;**132**(2):199-203

[9] Popper HH. Epithelioid cell granulomatosis of the lung: New insights and concepts. Sarcoidosis, Vasculitis, and Diffuse Lung Diseases. 1999;**16**(1):32-46

[10] Aubry MC. Necrotizing granulomatous inflammation: What does it mean if your special stains are negative? Modern Pathology. 2012;**25**:S31-S38. DOI: 10.1038/modpathol.2011.155

[11] Godman G, Churg J. Wegener's granulomatosis. A.M.A. Archives of Pathology. 1954;**58**:533-553. DOI: 10.1016/0002-9343(54)90255-7

[12] Yousem SA, Colby TV, Carrington CB. Lung biopsy in rheumatoid arthritis. The American Review of Respiratory Disease. 1985;**131**(5):770-777

[13] Yousem SA. The surgical pathology of pulmonary infarcts: Diagnostic confusion with granulomatous disease, vasculitis, and neoplasia. Modern Pathology. 2009;**22**:679-685. DOI: 10.1038/modpathol.2009.20

[14] Khmel'nitskij OK, Khmel'nitskaya NM. Pathomorphology of Human Mycosis. S.-Petersburg. Publishing House of S.Petersburg's Medical Academy of Postgraduate Education; 2005. p. 432

[15] Mukhopadhyay S, Gal AA. Granulomatous lung disease: An

approach to the differential diagnosis. Archives of Pathology & Laboratory Medicine. 2010;**134**:667-690

[16] Travis WD, Pittaluga S, Lipschik GY, et al. Atypical pathologic manifestations of Pneumocystis carinii pneumonia in the acquired immune deficiency syndrome: review of 123 lung biopsies from 76 patients with emphasis on cysts, vascular invasion, vasculitis, and granulomas. The American Journal of Surgical Pathology. 1990;**14**(7):615-625. DOI: 10.1097/00000478-199007000-00002

[17] Weber WR, Askin FB, Dehner LP. Lung biopsy in Pneumocystis carinii pneumonia: A histopathologic study of typical and atypical features. American Journal of Clinical Pathology. 1977;**67**(1):11-19. DOI: 10.1093/ajcp/67.1.11

[18] Flieder DB, Moran CA. Pulmonary dirofilariasis: A clinicopathologic study of 41 lesions in 39 patients. Human Pathology. 1999;**30**(3):251-256. DOI: 10.1016/s0046-8177(99)90001-1

[19] Strukov AI, Solov'eva IP. Tuberculosis Morphology in Modern Condition. Moscow: Medizina; 1976

[20] Corpe RF, Stergus I. Is the histopathology of nonphotochromogenic mycobacterial infections distinguishable from that caused by Mycobacterium tuberculosis? The American Review of Respiratory Disease. 1963;**87**:289-291

[21] Solovjeva IP, Batyrov FA, Ponomarev AB, Fedorov BT. Pathology of Tuberculosis and Differential Diagnostics of Granulomatous Diseases. Moscow: Atlas for the Post Graduation Education of Specialists of Scientific, Medical and Educational Institutions; 2005. p. 51

[22] Mukhopadhyay S, Farver CF, Vaszar LT, Dempsey OJ, Popper HH, Mani H, et al. Causes of pulmonary granulomas: A retrospective study of 500 cases from seven countries. Journal of Clinical Pathology. 2012;**65**:51-57. DOI: 10.1136/jclinpath-2011-200336

[23] Myers JL, Tazelaar HD. Challenges in pulmonary fibrosis: Problematic granulomatous lung disease. Thorax. 2008;**63**:78-84. DOI: 10.1136/thx.2004.031047

[24] Ulbright TM, Katzenstein AL. Solitary necrotizing granulomas of the lung: Differentiating features and etiology. The American Journal of Surgical Pathology. 1980;**4**(1):13-28. DOI: 10.1097/00000478-198002000-00002

Chapter 5

Clinical Manifestations of Sarcoidosis and Granulomatous Disorders

Suchibrata Das

Abstract

Sarcoidosis is a multisystem granulomatous disease, mainly involving the lungs, mediastinal and peripheral lymph nodes, liver, eyes, and skin. Cutaneous manifestations of sarcoid are variable and behave as "great imitators" of other cutaneous disorders. Cutaneous lesions are classified as specific and nonspecific forms. A large number of systemic sarcoidosis patients have specific cutaneous lesions, and this may be the presenting feature; isolated skin lesions may also present in some patients. Specific lesions of sarcoid are red-brown or red-violaceous in color, asymptomatic, and usually multiple in number. Different types of lesions may present in the same patient. This clinical appearance is due to the presence of epithelioid cell granulomas in the dermis.

Keywords: sarcoidosis, cutaneous sarcoidosis

1. Introduction

The granuloma is the result of interplay of an invading organism or antigen, chemical, drug or other irritant, prolonged antigenemia, macrophage activity, a Th1 cell response, B cell overactivity, circulating immune complexes, and a vast array of biological mediators [1]. Cutaneous granulomatosis can be localized or more disseminated, depending on their etiology. The typical lesion is a painless infiltrated papule, rounded, well limited, and reddish-pink and takes a yellowish color on diascopy, called apple-jelly. Its surface is smooth or slightly squamous, as there is generally no epidermal participation [2]. From a clinical point of view, it is useful to divide cutaneous granulomatosis into localized and more disseminated forms, although this distinction may sometimes be artificial. From a pathogenic point of view, they are divided into noninfectious and infectious granulomas [3].

2. Comprehensive classification of granulomatous disorders

A comprehensive classification of granulomatous disorders of the skin (according to American Academy of Dermatology, 76th Annual Meeting San Diego, CA USA) (**Table 1**) [4].

Noninfectious granulomatous disorders	Infectious granulomatous disorders
Epithelioid granulomas	*Caseating granulomas*
Sarcoidosis	Tuberculosis
Granulomatous rosacea/POD	Leprosy
Cutaneous Crohn's	Atypical mycobacterium
Orofacial granulomas	Leishmaniasis
Palisading granulomas	*Suppurative granulomas*
Granuloma annulare	Deep fungal
Elastolytic giant cell granuloma	Pyodermas
Necrobiosis lipoidica	Granulomatous STDs
Rheumatic nodules	
Reactive granulomatous disorders	
Xanthomatous granulomas	
Adult onset XG	
Adult onset APXG	
NXG	
Multicentric reticulohistiocytosis	
Rosai-Dorfman	
Xanthoma disseminatum	
Others	
Granulomatous vasculitis	
Lymphomatoid granulomatosis	
Foreign body reactions	
Granulomatous drug reactions	

Table 1.
Classification of granulomatous disorders of skin (American Academy of Dermatology, 76th Annual Meeting San Diego, CA USA).

3. Noninfectious granulomatous disorders

3.1 Epithelioid granulomas

3.1.1 Sarcoidosis

Sarcoidosis is a multiorgan disease. The most commonly affected organs are skin, lungs, and lymph nodes. Different epidemiological factors such as age, sex and race, the duration of the disease, and the sites of involvement affect the presentation of sarcoid. Cutaneous manifestations are extremely variable. Lesions of sarcoidosis are classified as "specific" (noncaseating granulomas are present in biopsy specimens of tissue) or "nonspecific" (lesions develop as a result of a reactive process without the formation of granulomas) [5].

Specific lesions develop in 9–15% of all sarcoidosis patients [5]. These lesions are highly variable in presentations and may be confused with many other skin diseases. The most frequent specific lesions are papules, plaques, lupus pernio, scar sarcoidosis, and subcutaneous sarcoidosis [5]. Erythema nodosum is the most common nonspecific lesion which develops in up to 25% of sarcoidosis cases [6]. Women are more commonly affected than men (W/M, 2:1) and black people than other ethnic groups [7].

The clinical appearance is due to the presence of epithelioid cell granulomas in the dermis. The epidermis rarely appears to be clinically involved [8]. Specific lesions are red-brown or red-violaceous in color and generally multiple and do not cause any symptoms which on diascopy reveals the brown-yellow or apple-jelly color, characteristics of granulomatous diseases. But it is usually more opaque than in lupus vulgaris [9]. Different types of cutaneous lesions may coexist in one patient.

3.1.1.1 Specific lesions of sarcoid

3.1.1.1.1 Maculopapular sarcoidosis

Lesions of maculopapular sarcoidosis are usually red-brown to purple in color and less than 1 cm in diameter. Sometimes they may be skin-colored, yellow-brown, or hypopigmented. They are slightly infiltrated, with little epidermal change. They are located on the face, particularly on the eyelids, around the orbits and the nasolabial folds, and on the scalp, occipital area of the neck, trunk, buttocks, and extremities (**Figure 1**). Lesions are commonly disseminated, and mucous membranes may even be involved [7, 9–11]. Diascopy shows the typical apple-jelly color characteristic of granulomatous skin lesions. These lesions are sometimes transient and appear to herald the onset of the disease [11]. Patients with papular lesions had a mean age of 47 years (9–83 years), and the usual duration of disease to heal is less than 2 years [12]. Acute organ involvement, such as sudden lymphadenopathy, acute arthritis, and acute uveitis abnormal chest radiographs, has been associated with this type of

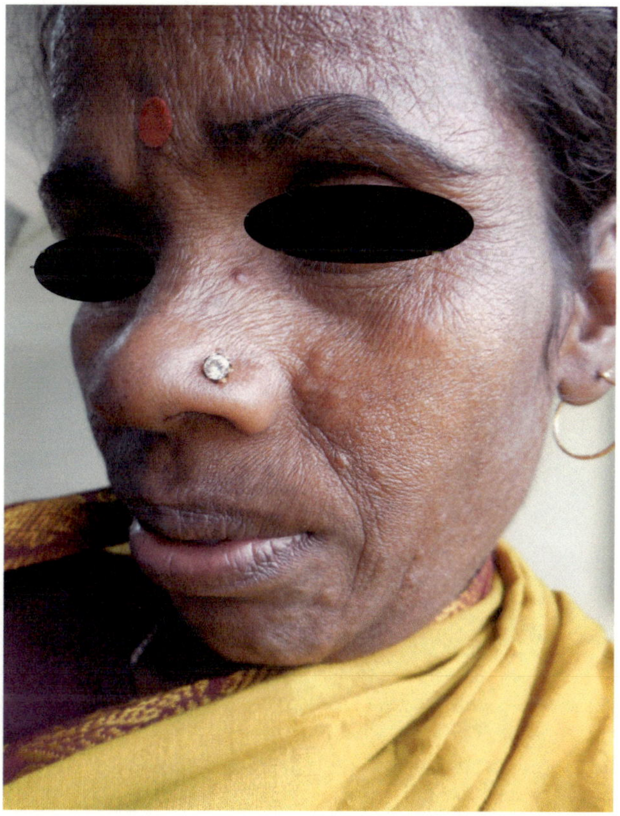

Figure 1.
Papular sarcoid.

eruption [9]. The intrathoracic involvement occurs in the early stage of the disease, bilateral hilar lymphadenopathy with or without parenchymal infiltration (up to stage II) (60%), and lymphadenopathy in 50% of the patients [13].

3.1.1.1.2 Nodular and plaque sarcoid

It more commonly develops on the back, buttocks, face, and extensor surfaces of the extremities [7]. It is as common as maculopapular sarcoid [10]. It is usually present as multiple round or oval, infiltrated reddish-brown plaques [7, 10], larger than 10 mm in diameter, more indurated, thicker, and persistent than papular sarcoid (**Figure 2**). Sometimes it is mammillated and can be associated with nodular dermal lesions [14]. More than 90% of cases are chronic with disease activity persisting after 2 years [12].

3.1.1.1.3 Lupus pernio

It is the characteristic cutaneous manifestation of sarcoidosis [15]. Lupus pernio refers primarily to diffuse, violaceous to telangiectatic plaque lesions of the nose, cheeks, ears, and fingers [16–19] (**Figure 3**). It tends to appear in older people, especially the black women affected more frequently [20, 21]. The lesions enlarge and become confluent to form progressively disfiguring nodular plaques on the nose and adjacent cheeks [21]. The lesions can involve the upper respiratory tract and cause nasal ulceration, obstruction, and perforation of the nasal septum [15, 22, 23]. Some cases have developed plaques on the arms, thighs, and buttocks [21, 24] and sausage-shaped expansion of the phalanges [16, 25]. This form of sarcoidosis can be recalcitrant to systemic corticosteroids and other immune-suppressants and may be an indicator of current or impending organ involvement [24]. Also it usually follows an extremely chronic course—2–25 years in published series [11, 13].

3.1.1.1.4 Scar sarcoid

Scar sarcoid presents as erythematous, cutaneous, or subcutaneous swelling in the area of an old scar or beside a scar and the development of papules and nodules within the original scars [26]. Scar sarcoidosis can occur on skin sites damaged by a range of factors, including mechanical injuries, venipuncture,

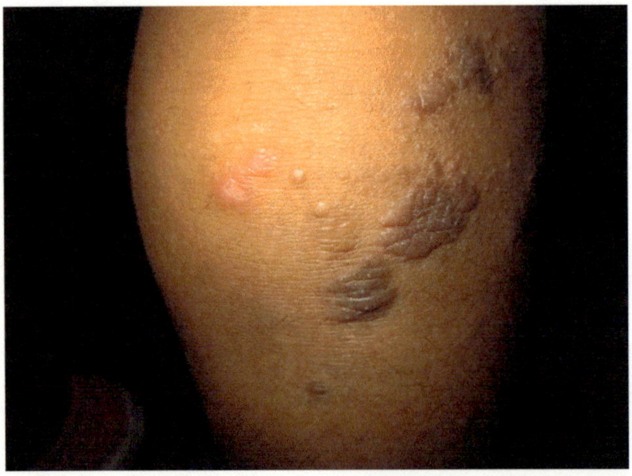

Figure 2.
Plaque sarcoid.

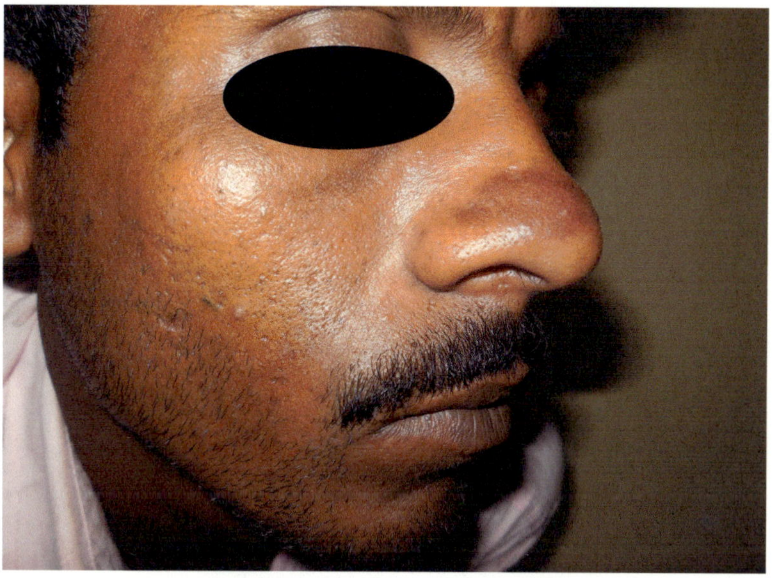

Figure 3.
Lupus pernio.

intramuscular injections, inoculations, tattoos, and infections such as herpes zoster [27] (**Figure 4**). Foreign material within the scar, deposited by external factors including those stated above, is a possible cause of epithelioid granuloma [28]. The specific skin lesions that occur and the resulting sarcoidosis may be associated with the severity and duration of the disease, with scar sarcoidosis often being accompanied by systemic involvement [29]. Alterations, such as further damage or stress to the existing scars, often prompt worsening of sarcoidosis [30]. Scar sarcoidosis can appear at the onset of disease and must be looked for whenever a diagnosis of sarcoid is considered [8]. However, more commonly it is associated with longstanding pulmonary and mediastinal involvement, uveitis, peripheral lymphadenopathy, bony cyst, and parotid infiltration [9, 11].

3.1.1.1.5 Subcutaneous sarcoid (Darier-Roussy sarcoid)

Peak incidence of subcutaneous sarcoid is the fourth decade of life; females are more affected than male; these are asymptomatic to slightly tender subcutaneous lesions typically involving the upper extremities. Majority lessons are erythematous (57%), followed by skin colored (30%), hypopigmented, or violaceous [7, 10] (**Figure 5**). Lesions are usually multiple, clustered, and bilaterally asymmetrical [32]. There are autoimmune disease associations in a subset of patients. There is strong association with a systemic disease component at the outset of disease, notably bilateral hilar adenopathy; noninfectious panicular sarcoidal or epithelioid granulomas with minimal lymphocytic inflammation; and a favorable response to oral corticosteroid therapy [31].

3.1.1.1.6 Less common form of cutaneous sarcoidosis

A wide variety of different cutaneous manifestations have been reported, and the clinical pictures are highly heterogeneous.

Annular sarcoid. Annular lesions are well-recognized forms of cutaneous sarcoidosis, amounting to around 8% of all skin lesions according to a recent study

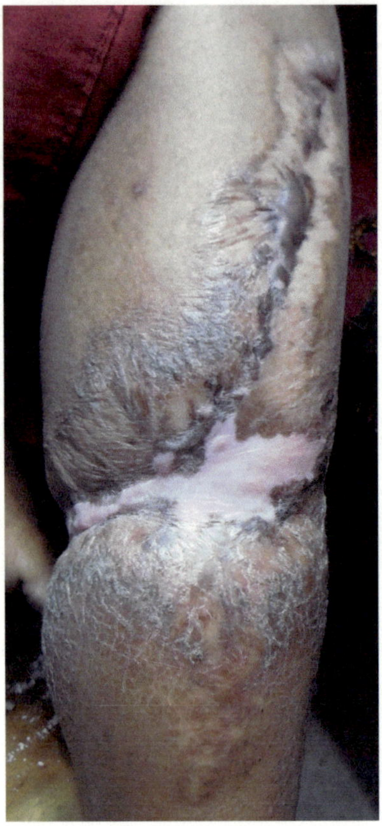

Figure 4.
Scar sarcoid.

from India [32]. Papular lesions may coalesce or be arranged in annular patterns, usually with a red-brown hue. Lesions are indurated, have central clearing with hypopigmentation, and atrophy and scarring may occur (**Figure 6**). Usually, the photo-exposed areas that are affected have a predilection for the face, forehead, and neck. Alopecia may occur in the center of the lesions [32, 33].

Angiolupoid sarcoidosis. Angiolupoid sarcoidosis is an infrequent variant of the disease, affecting 8% of patients with cutaneous sarcoidosis [32]. It manifests clinically as single plaques with central hypopigmentation, which eventually acquire annular shape with prominent telangiectasias, preferentially located on the face, ears, or scalp [32] (**Figure 7**). It is usually present in women [34]. The cutaneous manifestation may be the first sign of a systemic sarcoidosis with the lung (stage 2) and gland involvement that are refractory to several conventional drug therapies [34].

Hypopigmented sarcoid. Dermal nodules with surrounding hypopigmentation and macular hypopigmented areas occur predominantly on the limbs. They may be tender but have no associated anesthesia [35].

In the nodules, the pigment is retained in the center where the color is dark red-brown. The lesions are ill-defined, and perifollicular pigment is usually retained at the periphery. Nodules are unattached to underlying structures and tender when pressed or squeezed [35]. Sarcoid granuloma present in all nodules but in half of macules [36].

Morphea-like lesions. Clinical features are indistinguishable from those of true morphea, and the cutaneous lesions may precede or arise years after the extracutaneous sarcoidosis [37]. Lesions are coalescing hyperpigmented atrophic plaques, may be indurated, usually in limbs, mainly lower limbs [38] (**Figure 8**).

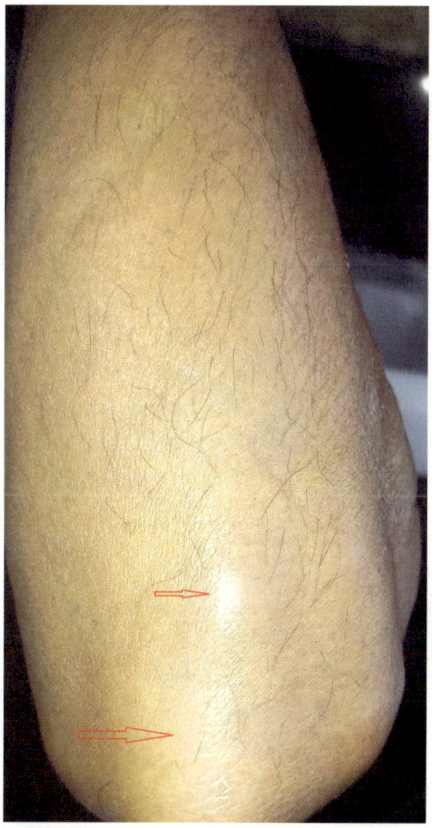

Figure 5.
Subcutaneous sarcoidosis.

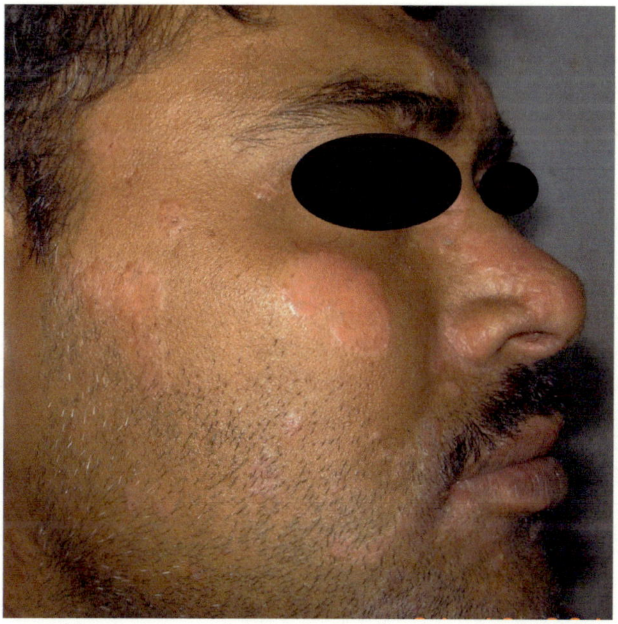

Figure 6.
Annular sarcoid.

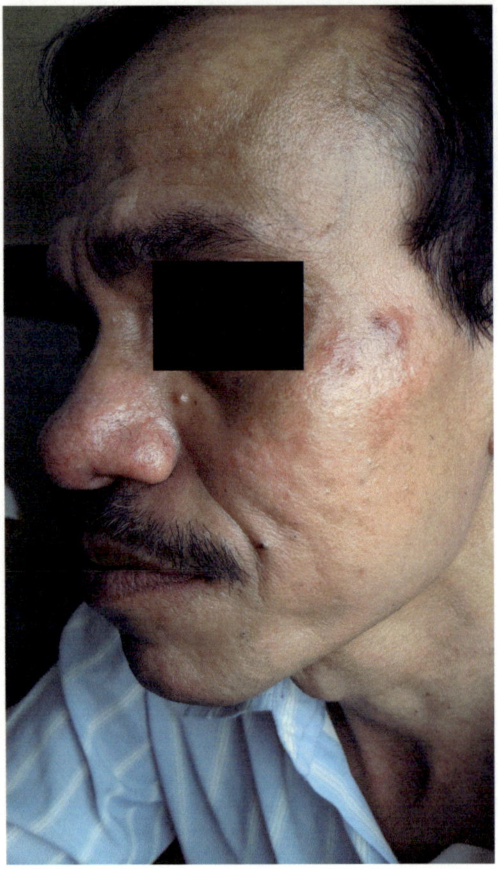

Figure 7.
Angiolupoid sarcoid.

Psoriasiform sarcoidosis. It is a rare morphologic manifestation of sarcoidosis. The appearance of its lesion are psoriasiform and infiltrated (**Figure 9**); some were annular, and others followed the natural lines of cleavage of the skin [39]. This type of sarcoidosis is usually peculiar to the dark skin [40].

Lichenoid sarcoidosis. About 1–2% of all cases of skin sarcoidosis are in this variety. It is characterized by abundant pinhead-sized yellowish lesions closely grouped in round or oval clusters, slightly scaling, mimicking lichen planus [41]. Lesions can occasionally show superficial scaling (**Figure 10a, b**). Sites commonly involved include trunk, limbs, and face [42]. It appears symmetrically and in crops and is associated with the eye and joint complications [41, 43]. The dermoscopy findings usually reveal circular or oval yellowish brown lesions with the absence of Wickham's striae. This feature is not specific for sarcoidosis, but such homogeneous appearance of lesions indicates a granulomatous skin disease [44].

Ulcerative sarcoidosis. Ulcerative sarcoidosis usually develops from the papulonodular sarcoid lesions by ulceration, but some arose de novo. Ulcers also developed in psoriasiform, atrophie, lymphedematous, erythrodermic, verrucous, suppurative, and elephantine lesions [45]. Lesions usually occur in the lower limb, and the upper limb may also be affected; sometimes lesions are generalized [45, 46]. Ulcers tended to heal with scarring [46] (**Figure 11**). Women are affected three times more than men, and blacks are affected slightly more than whites. Ulcer is a presenting feature in nearly 30% of patients, half of them having an initial lesion of other types [45], and cutaneous lesions are usually the presenting sign of sarcoidosis [45].

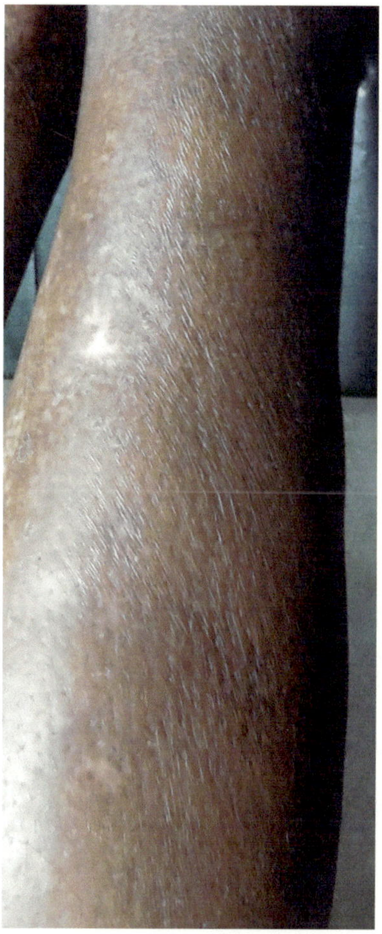

Figure 8.
Morpheaform sarcoidosis.

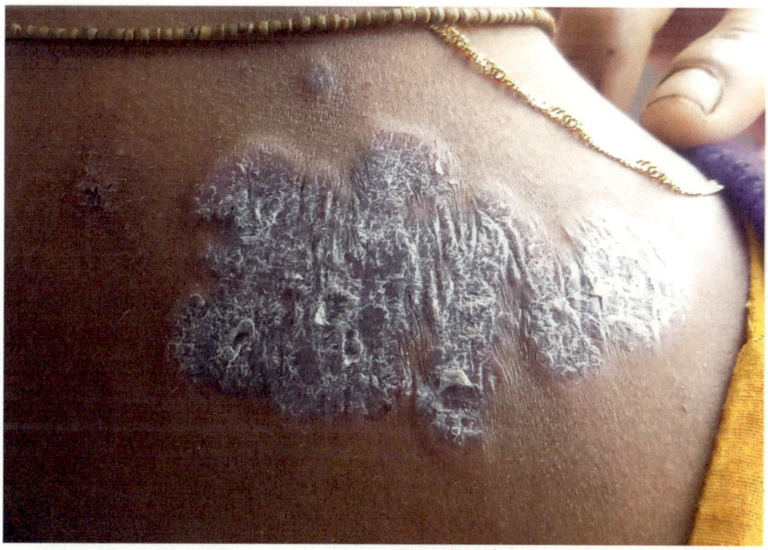

Figure 9.
Psoriasisform sarcoidosis.

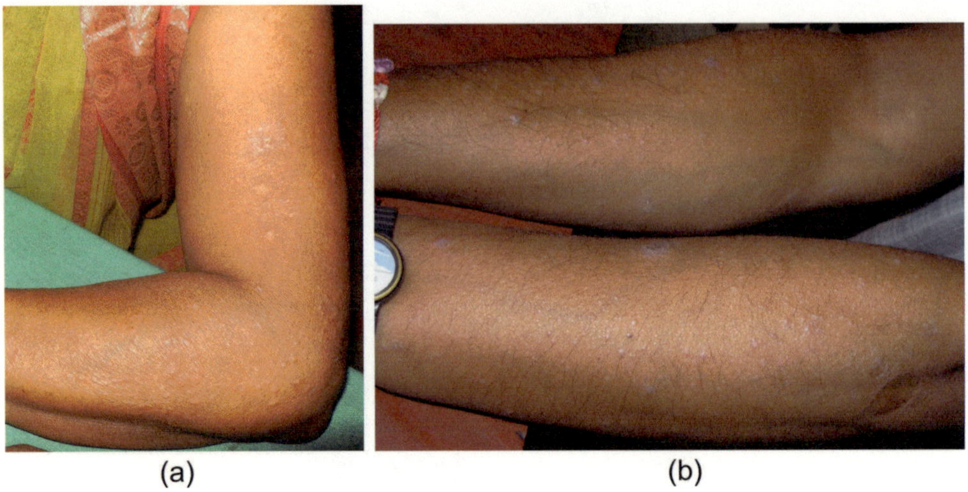

Figure 10.
(a and b) Lichenoid sarcoidosis.

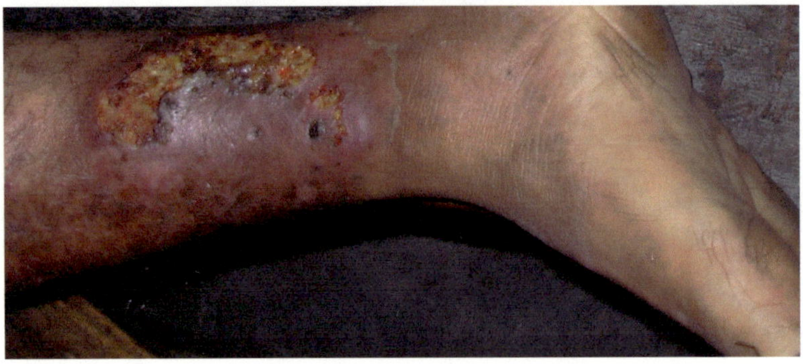

Figure 11.
Ulcerative sarcoidosis.

Verrucous sarcoidosis. All reported patients of verrucous sarcoidosis have been of African descent with a longstanding systemic disease. Usually, systemic sarcoidosis of other internal organs is present [47]. Lesions may be multiple exophytic, extensively verrucous yellowish-to-whitish lesions with a reddish-brown circinate border, size ranging from 1.0 to 2.0 cm in diameter [48].

3.1.1.2 Nonspecific lesions of sarcoid

Erythema nodosum, the most common nonspecific lesion, develops in 20–25% of sarcoidosis cases [6, 49]. Frequently, it is the initial manifestation of disease. It is the marker of acute and benign sarcoidosis and tends to affect younger people than infiltrative cutaneous lesions [12]. Sarcoidosis is the second most common cause of erythema nodosum [50]. If sarcoid is associated with EN, it usually runs a benign and self-limited course [51]. Women are affected three to six times more frequently than men [52]. EN can occur in all age groups, but it is typically seen between the second and fourth decades of life. The higher prevalence of erythema nodosum among young people is considered to be due to the higher incidence of sarcoidosis in this age group [11]. EN is characterized by sudden onset of symmetric, tender, erythematous, warm nodules and raised plaques, usually located on the shins, ankles, and knees (**Figure 12**). Nodules are from 1 to 5 cm or more in diameter and

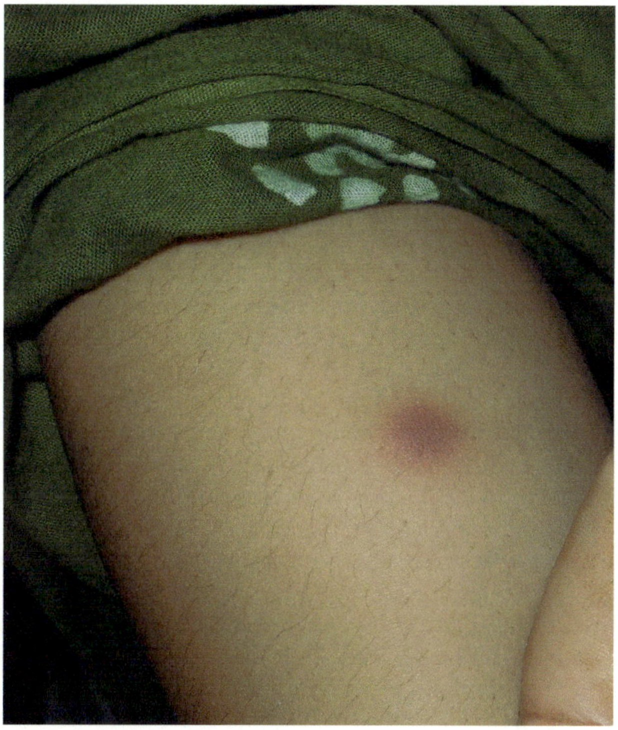

Figure 12.
Erythema nodosum.

distributed bilaterally. Nodules may become confluent, resulting in erythematous plaques. In rare instances, more extensive lesions may appear, involving the thighs, extensor aspects of the arms, the neck, and even the face. Initially the nodules are bright red in color; within a few days, they become flat, with a livid red or purplish color and finally a yellow or greenish appearance, often taking on the look of a deep bruise (erythema contusiformis). This contusiformis color evolution is quite characteristic of erythema nodosum and allows a specific diagnosis in late-stage lesions [53]. Ulceration is never seen in erythema nodosum, and the nodules heal without atrophy or scarring [54]. Usually, acute bouts of erythema nodosum are associated with a fever of 38–39°C, fatigue, malaise, arthralgia, headache, abdominal pain, vomiting, cough, or diarrhea. Episcleral lesions and phlyctenular conjunctivitis may also accompany the cutaneous lesions. Less frequent clinical manifestations associated with erythema nodosum are lymphadenopathy, hepatomegaly, splenomegaly, and pleuritis [55]. Eruption generally lasts from 3 to 6 weeks, but persistence beyond this time is not unusual. Recurrences are not uncommon. Erythema nodosum in children has a much shorter duration than in adults, arthralgias are seen in a minority of the patients, and fever is an accompanying manifestation in fewer than half of the cases [56].

Another nonspecific lesion of sarcoid is Lofgren's syndrome, an acute form of sarcoidosis characterized by erythema nodosum, bilateral hilar lymphadenopathy (BHL), and symmetric polyarthritis [57]. Arthritis in sarcoidosis is usually symmetrical; the ankles are involved in more than 90% of the cases; the knees, small joints of the hands or feet, wrists, and elbows are involved in 15–40% [58–60]. Local pain, soft-tissue swelling, periarticular tenderness, edema, and joint effusion may be present [61]. In 1953, Lofgren characterized 212 adult patients of bilateral hilar lymphadenopathy who were practically regarded as having sarcoidosis based on the absence of tuberculosis. Lofgren demonstrated that EN was present at the onset of the disease in 113 cases in which articular symptoms were common (101 cases, 89%). There was either pain only in the joints (20%) or pain accompanied by swelling (69%) [62]. Lofgren's syndrome was regarded as a self-limiting disease that is generally resolved within the first year, with the mean duration ranging from 3 weeks to 3.7 months [57, 60]. However, 8% of patients had active symptoms 2 years after the onset; 6% had episodes of recurrent sarcoidosis 2.20 years after the diagnosis [62].

3.1.2 Granulomatous rosacea

Granulomatous rosacea is a distinct variant of rosacea. Lewandowsky described the "rosacea-like tuberculid" as having a clinical appearance similar to that of a papular form of rosacea; however, it appeared as yellow-brown "apple-jelly" nodules on diascopy and as tuberculoid granulomas on histologic examination [63]. Later it was noted that granulomas can be seen in typical rosacea [64]. Thus rosacea may be manifested by a clinical and a histologic spectrum that includes granuloma formation in some patients [65]. Lesions are persistent, firm, and non-tender; red to brown papule or nodule arises primarily on otherwise normal appearing skin around the mouth and eyes and on the cheeks [66] (**Figure 13**). Granulomatous rosacea often does not present facial erythema, is not limited to facial convexities, often has periocular lesions, and shows an asymmetrical distribution [67]. Some studies have demonstrated that patients with this variant present clinically with monomorphic yellow-brown and red papules or nodules situated predominantly over the cheeks and periorificial areas [68, 69]. Although clinical correlation is important, the diagnosis of GR is dependent upon the histopathologic finding of a granulomatous infiltrate [70, 71].

3.1.3 Cutaneous Crohn's disease

Skin manifestations of Crohn's disease (CD) have been classified into three principal classes: granulomatous or CD specific, reactive, and secondary to nutritional deficiency [72]. CD-specific lesions account for the majority of lesions

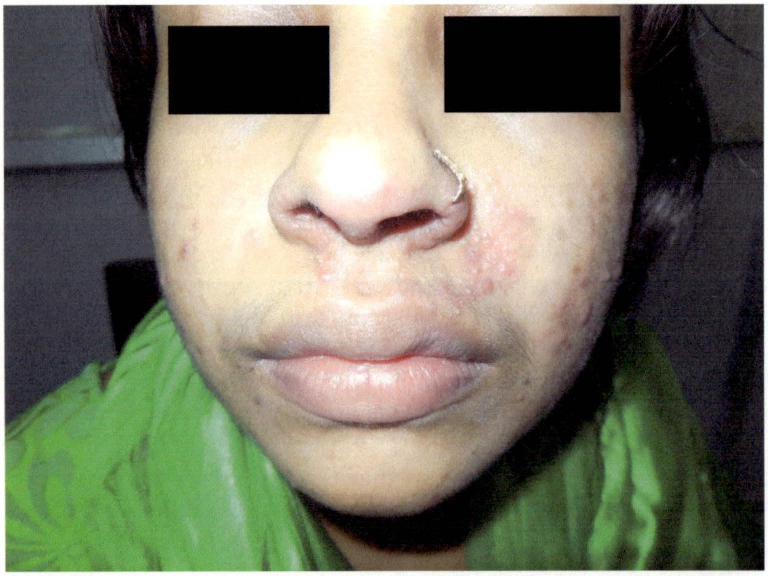

Figure 13.
Granulomatous rosacea.

observed. The best recognized are perianal and peristomal fissures and fistulae and oral disease [73]. Skin lesions commonly complicate CD with reported prevalence rates as high as 44% [74–76]. The characteristic lesions of metastatic Crohn's diseases are erythematous plaques and nodules and cutaneous ulceration. Secondary features like scale or crust may present [73] (**Figure 14**). Lesions involving intertriginous and genital skin usually ulcerate, owing to friction [77]. Lesions may be solitary or multiple, usually asymptomatic, but may be tender on palpation [77]. The oral manifestation of CD in the buccal mucosa is cobblestoning, while the gingival and alveolar mucosae often have tiny nodules. Linear ulcers are more common in sulci. The lips may become swollen, hardened, or ulcerated, especially at the angles of the mouth [78]. Genital lesions are the most common presentation of MCD in children; 85% of the cases present with swelling and/or induration of the genitals with or without erythema. In adults, the most frequent lesions are nodules and plaques, with or without ulceration on the arms and legs, followed by ulcers on the genitals [77].

3.1.4 Orofacial granulomatosis

The term orofacial granulomatosis (OFG) includes a group of disorders showing chronic, noncaseating granulomatous lesions involving the perioral tissue of the face and oral mucosa [79]. Possible systemic diseases, such as tuberculosis, sarcoidosis, and other diseases with the same clinical findings are to be excluded before to diagnose orofacial granuloma [80]. Clinically, OFG generally presents as swelling of upper and/lower lip, even the whole orofacial region including the chin, cheeks, periorbital and zygomatic tissues, eyelids, and forehead, unilaterally or bilaterally, either alone or in combination, though classic presentation is that of a non-tender recurrent labial swelling that may eventually become persistent [79] (**Figure 15**). Furthermore, manifestations include angular cheilitis, mucosal ulcerations, vertical fissures of the lips, mucosal tags, and lingua plicata [81]. However, the clinical

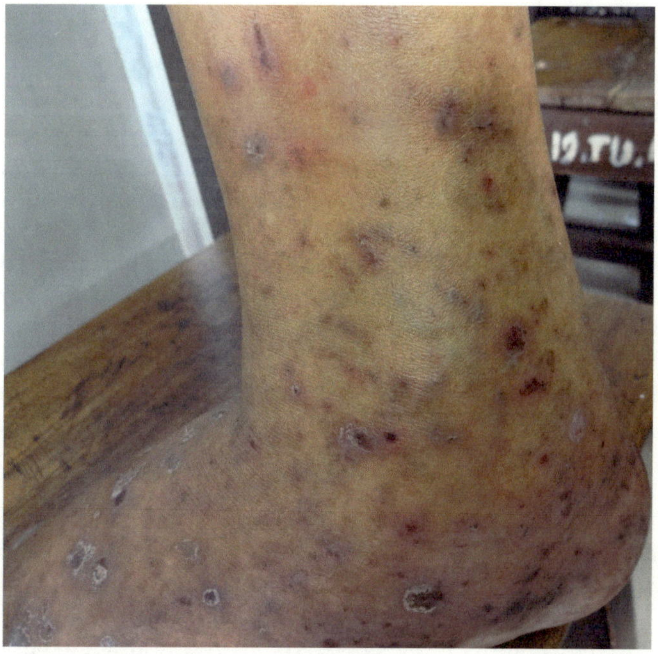

Figure 14.
Metastatic Crohn's disease.

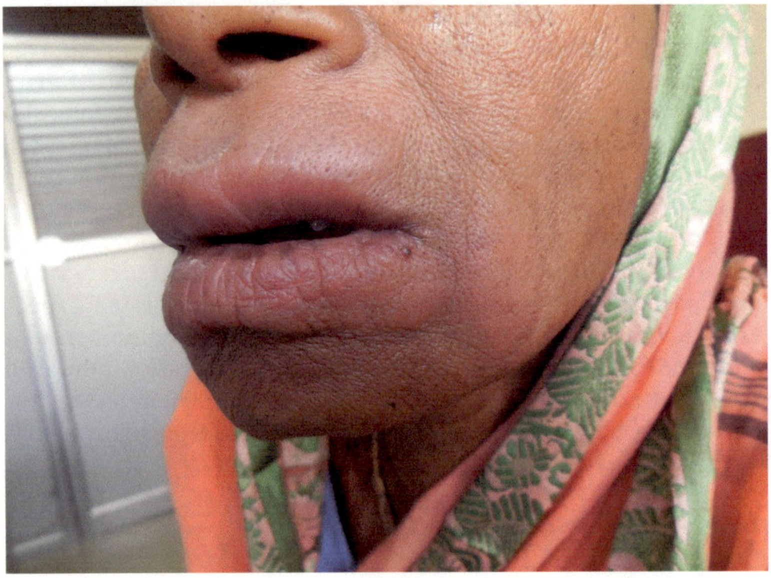

Figure 15.
Orofacial Granulomatosis.

presentation can be highly variable, making the diagnosis difficult to establish, i.e., intraoral involvement may take the form of hypertrophy, erythema, or nonspecific erosions involving the gingiva, oral mucosa, or tongue [80–82]. Clinicopathological correlation is required for final diagnosis.

3.2 Palisading granulomas

3.2.1 Granuloma annulare

It is characterized by ringed erythematous plaques with granulomatous inflammation seen histologically. There are four clinical variants of GA-localized, generalized, or disseminated, subcutaneous, and perforating [83].

The localized, commonest variety, nearly three-fourths of all GA cases, is in this group. Lesions are usually present as skin-colored or erythematous papules, without epidermal change, that are often arranged in arciform or annular patterns, usually less than 5 cm in diameter, and enlarge centrifugally [84–86] (**Figure 16**). Subcutaneous and superficial papular lesions may coexist in some patients, particularly in children [84]. The number of lesions may be single or multiple, in equal distribution. The commonest site of involvement is the hands and arms (63%), lower extremity in 20%, trunk alone in 5%, and all extremities affected in 7% of patients. Both sexes are equally affected [84]. Lesions are temporary in 70% of cases. In 51%, clearing happens within 2 years. The age of the patients did not affect the prognosis to any great extent, and usually three-fourths of patients recover [84].

In generalized (disseminated) granuloma annulare, innumerable number of lesions, arranged in symmetrical distribution, presents in any part of the body, but the face and also the palm and sole are usually spared. There may be macules, papules, or nodules [84], arranged in an annular fashion [86]; colors range from skin-tone to red, yellow, or tan. There is controversy about generalized and disseminated GA. In original description, granuloma annulare was defined as

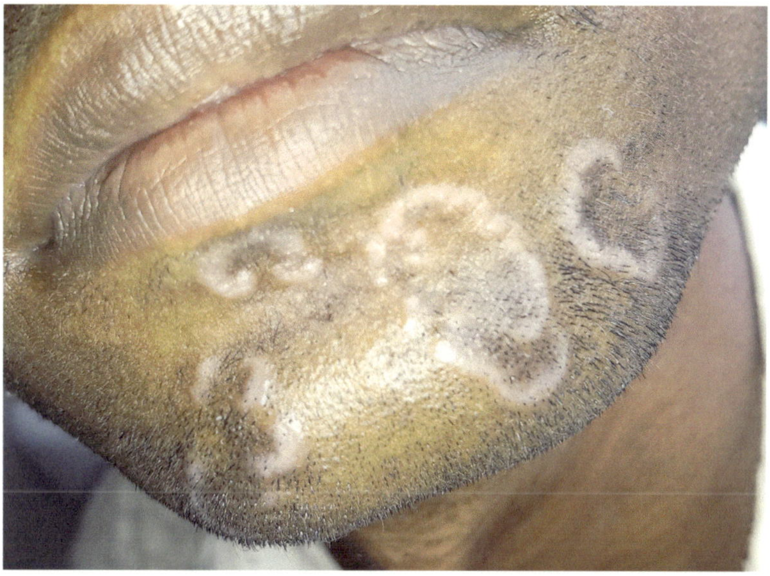

Figure 16.
Granuloma annulare.

generalized involvement of at least the trunk and the upper or lower extremities [86] (**Figure 17a, b**). It is asymptotic and usually persists for 3–4 years but may persist up to 10 years and recur [84]. The age of onset is bimodal in distribution, with 80% of patients presenting in the fourth to seventh decades and the remainder presenting before the age of 10 [84]. Female to male ratio is slightly higher [86].

Subcutaneous granuloma annulare, also known as pseudorheumatoid nodule, is a self-limiting disorder usually found between the ages of 3 and 6 years, and the sex ratio is 1:1 [84, 87, 88]. They are small, pinkish, asymptomatic, hard-elastic, nodular, isolated lesions, or associated with local annular granuloma. The overlying skin is healthy. Sites include the pretibial region, elbow, forearm, forehead, scalp, and dorsal surfaces of the hands and feet [84] (**Figure 18**). Lesions situated on the head adhere to the periosteum and are fixed with respect to the underlying layers, whereas those on the extremities adhere to the fascia and are therefore mobile [84, 89].

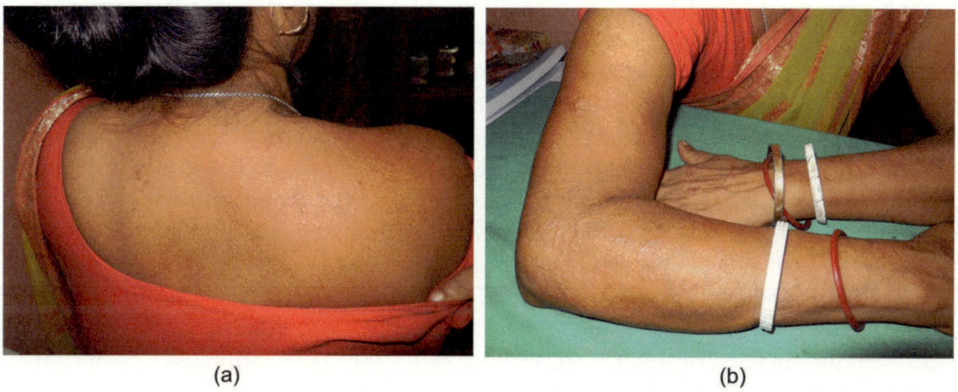

Figure 17.
(a and b) Generalized granuloma annulare.

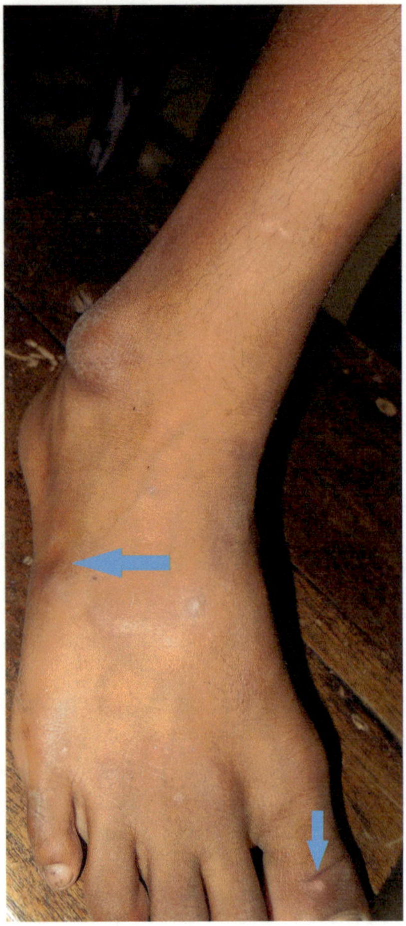

Figure 18.
Subcutaneous granuloma annulare.

3.2.2 Annular elastolytic giant cell granuloma

It is usually a disease of middle-aged, Caucasian women [90]. Onset is sudden but progressive, and varying in duration from 1 month to 10 years [91]. Clinically, AEGCG presents as multiple, large, annular plaques with a raised, erythematous border and central atrophy. The lesions are mostly located on sun-exposed areas such as the face and neck, but they are also seen on nonexposed skin although rare reports of a papular variant of AEGCG exist [92, 93]. It is currently unclear whether they simply represent a variant of granuloma annulare occurring on sun-damaged skin or distinct disease. There are two patterns. One is a single, asymptomatic, atrophic-appearing, yellow thin plaque on forehead, and the other is multiple, upper extremity, and trunk lesions occurring mainly on sun-exposed areas predominantly in women (**Figure 19**). A papular and arciform variant is also described [90, 91]. The histopathologic features are best demonstrated by a biopsy of the elevated edge of the plaque [94]. The lesions may persist for months to years resolving with either mottled pigmentation or normal-appearing skin [95]. Association with temporal arteritis is reported [96]. There have been reported cases of AEGCG associated with diabetes, sarcoidosis, and hematological malignancies [97, 98]. Patient of AEGCG may associate with Barrett's esophagus. The patient had hepatic nodules that showed nonspecific granulomas with elastolysis, similar to the skin lesions [99].

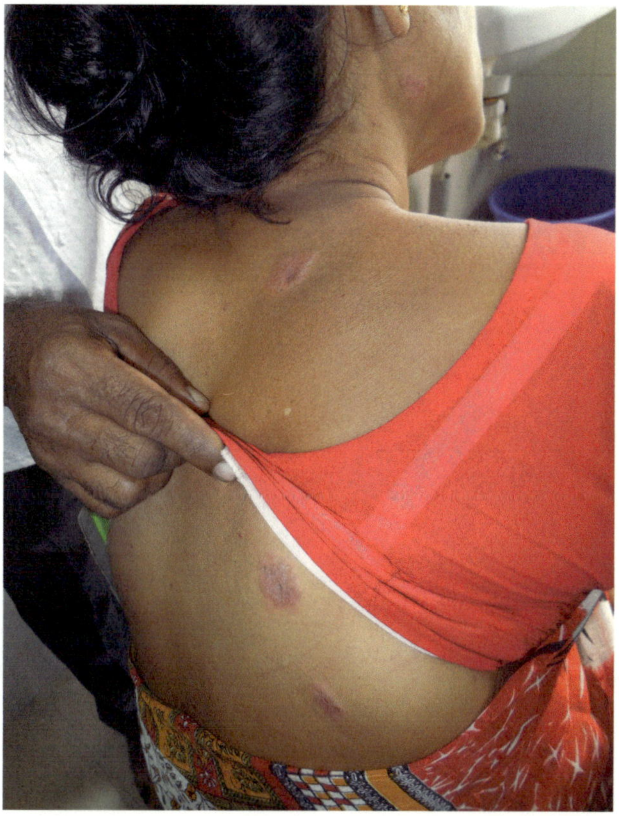

Figure 19.
Annular elastolytic giant cell granuloma.

3.2.3 Necrobiosis lipoidica

Necrobiosis lipoidica developed in the fourth decade of life and, in type 1 diabetes mellitus, in the third decade [100, 101]. Females are more affected than male (3:1). It is rare in childhood. NL is usually present on bilateral lower extremities, typically pretibial skin, but face, scalp, trunk, groin, and upper extremities can also be affected.

It forms as well-circumscribed papules and nodules with active erythematous borders that slowly coalesce into plaques. The plaques appear violaceous and contain a central area that initially appears red-brown but later progresses to a yellow-brown discoloration with atrophic, waxy appearance with prominent telangiectatic vessels [102]. But this classical presentation may not present in Indian patients where common presentation is erythematous plaque [103] (**Figure 20**). Lesions are 1–3 in number [102]. They are usually asymptomatic but may be painful or hypoesthetic or anesthetic [104]. NL lesions can also exhibit the Koebner phenomenon. Up to one-thirds of the patients with NL may develop ulcerations secondary to minor trauma [100]. Occasional reports of squamous cell carcinoma arising in areas of long-term lesions have also been reported [105].

3.2.4 Rheumatoid nodule

Rheumatoid nodules are commonly found in patients with rheumatoid arthritis as later manifestation of active arthritic disease [106]. It occurs as subcutaneous nodules;

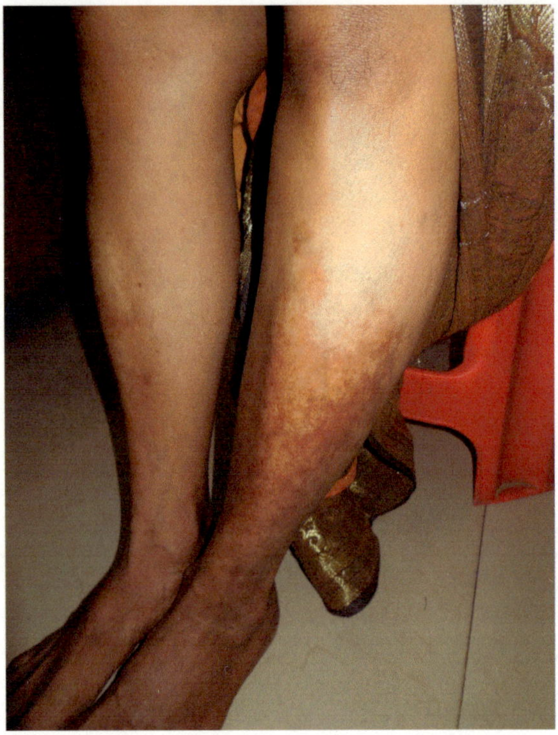

Figure 20.
Necrobiosis lipoidica.

the most common extra-articular feature of RA [107, 108] is present in about 25–42% [107, 108] of RA patients, although similar nodules have been observed in nonrheumatoid conditions, such as granuloma annulare and necrobiosis lipoidica [109]. Nodules are skin colored, can be solitary or multiple, and range from <5 mm to many centimeters in diameter [106] (**Figure 21**). They lie deeply subcutaneously and can adhere to underlying periosteum, tendons, or bursae, although others may be epidermal and freely movable [110]. Most are firm and painless and often go unnoticed by the average patient, but those found on the plantar surfaces of the feet or palms may feel uncomfortable [110].

3.2.5 Reactive granulomatous disorders

Reactive granulomatous disorders are reactive granulomatous processes, which present with a cutaneous granulomatous eruptions in response to medications, autoimmune disease, arthritides, and internal malignancies. There is a wide spectrum of clinical morphologic patterns and a broad array of histologic subtypes that may occur. The common RGDs are palisaded neutrophilic and granulomatous dermatitis (PNGD), interstitial granulomatous dermatitis (IGD), and interstitial granulomatous drug reaction (IGDR) [111].

The classic clinical presentation of PNGD is that of flesh-colored to erythematous papules, which may be umbilicated or crusted, appearing symmetrically on the extremities particularly around the elbows [112–114] (**Figure 22**). Palisaded neutrophilic and granulomatous dermatitis is seen in association with a number of systemic diseases. The diseases most commonly reported with PNGD include connective tissue diseases—particularly systemic lupus erythematosus—as well as inflammatory arthritis, hematologic disorders, and rarely infections or medications [111]. Patients

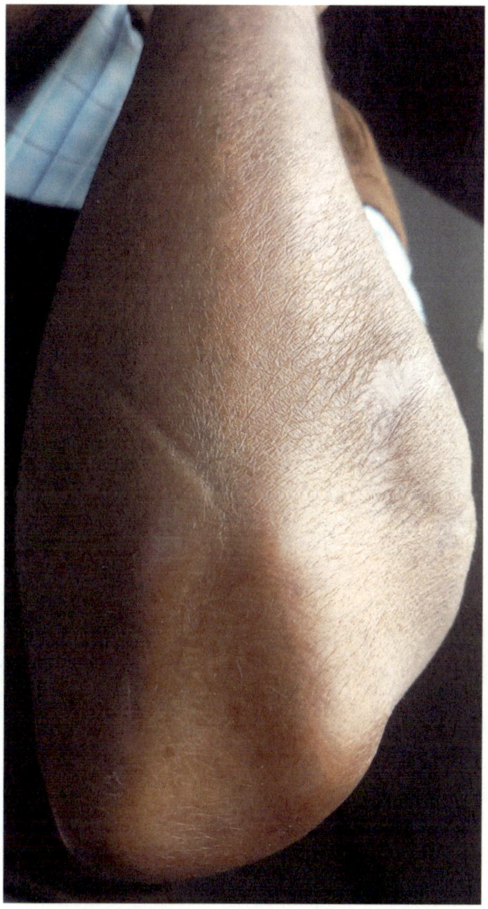

Figure 21.
Rheumatoid nodule.

of all ages may develop PNGD, although reports in childhood are rare [114]. Women are affected more frequently (approximately 3:1 ratio), likely owing to the systemic diseases associated with PNGD [114].

In interstitial granulomatous dermatitis (IGD), the initial description was linear subcutaneous cords or bands on the proximal trunk [115], and also erythematous to violaceous patches or plaques symmetrically on the upper trunk and proximal limbs are a frequent manifestation [116]. IGD is generally seen in the setting of an underlying systemic disease, similar to PNGD [111].

There is contradiction whether interstitial granulomatous drug reaction (IGDR) is another entity or subtype of interstitial granulomatous dermatitis [111]. The classic description of IGDR is erythematous to violaceous plaques, often annular, concentrated on the inner arms, proximal medial thighs, proximal trunk, and intertriginous sites, with distinctive histologic features [117].

3.3 Xanthomatous granulomas

3.3.1 Adult-onset xanthogranuloma

Xanthogranuloma (XG) is the most common non-Langerhans cell histiocytosis, which usually occurs in the early part of life [118]. It is rare in adults, usually occurring in the third and fourth decades of life [119].

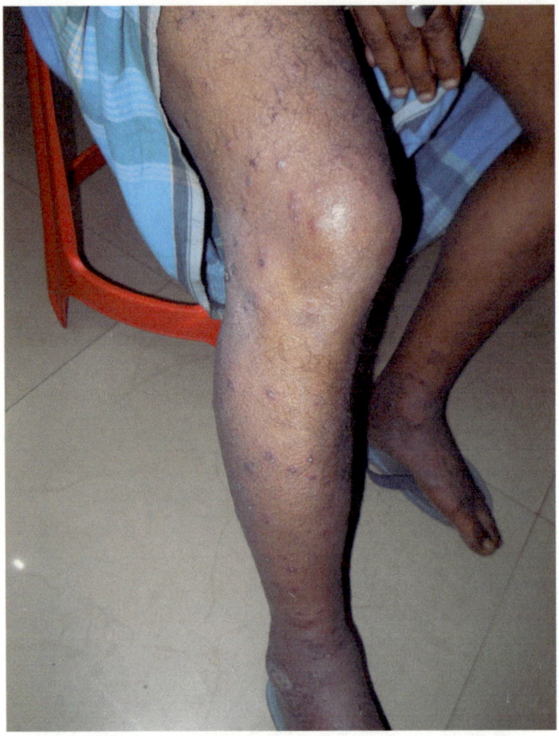

Figure 22.
Palisaded neutrophilic and granulomatous dermatitis.

Lesions of XG are usually orange or erythematous-brown papule nodule [120], varying the tonality with the age of the lesions [118]. XGA usually occurs as a single lesion in 2/3 of cases located on the face but may be seen in the trunk or limbs [119, 121].

There are three recognized main clinical forms of adult onset xanthogranuloma: a small nodular/papular (2–5 mm); large nodular (5–20 mm); and giant xanthogranuloma (more than 20 mm [122]). Multiple adult onset xanthogranuloma is defined when there are more than five XG lesions. It appears to be more common among men [121].

3.3.2 Adult onset asthma with periorbital xanthogranuloma (adult onset APXG)

Adult onset asthma with periorbital granuloma (AAPOX) syndrome was first described in 1993 by Jakobiec et al. and is considered to be a periorbital disease with a specific granulomatous inflammation [123, 124].

Skin surrounding the orbit is yellow-orange in color, with swelling of mainly upper and also lower eyelid with compromised eyelid movement. There is associated allergic sinusitis and adult onset asthma [125].

3.3.3 Necrobiotic xanthogranuloma

It is a chronic, progressive granulomatous disorder with cutaneous and extracutaneous involvement. The mean age is 61.6 years [126]. The mean (SD) age at presentation was 61.6 (14.2) years; females are more commonly affected (62.6%) than male. Most patients are white (87%) [126]. More than one site is usually involved [127].

It usually manifests as yellowish or yellow-orange, red or brown papules, plaques, and nodules [126]. The commonest site of involvement is the periorbital area [128]. Trunk [127] and also the extremities [126] are the second most common site.

Dermatologic symptoms may present up to 60% of patients such as itching, burning, tenderness, and pain. Nearly half of patients may ulcerate, the most common secondary feature [126, 127].

3.3.4 Multicentric reticulohistiocytosis

It is a rare histiocytic proliferative disease in which joints, skin, mucous membranes, and internal organs are affected [129]. Onset is usually insidious; cutaneous manifestations usually follow the articular signs and symptoms [130].

The peak occurrence is seen in middle age with the average age of 40–50 years at presentation, but MRH can present at any age [131–133].

The classic skin lesions are firm brown or yellow papule and plaque. Extensor surfaces are predominantly affected, particularly on the hands and forearm, and also the face, scalp, hands, and ears are often affected, but involvement of lower trunk and legs is rare. Coral bead-like lesions may occur around the nail folds which may lead to nail dystrophy. The size varies from a few millimeters to centimeters [134]. Lesions in proximity to joints may be largely nodular. Lesions may ulcerate. The vermicular erythematous lesions around the nostrils are thought to be a characteristic of MRH [135]. Mucosal lesions present from 30 to 50% patients [131, 133], oral and nasal mucosa are the frequently involved sites, but lesions may be distributed along the lips, buccal mucosa, tongue, and gingival and nasal septum. Usually lesions are asymptomatic; around 25% patients complain of pruritus.

3.3.5 Rosai-Dorfman syndrome

The hallmark of Rosai-Dorfman disease is massive cervical lymphadenopathy. Other lymph node groups like axillary, inguinal, and mediastinal nodes may also be affected. In about 10% of patients, the cutaneous manifestations present, which are asymptomatic xanthoma-like, yellowish, or reddish-brown papules, nodules, and plaques which may ulcerate [136]. Involvement of extra-nodal sites like the nasal cavity, paranasal sinuses, eyelids, orbit, skeletal system, salivary glands, and central nervous system has been reported [137, 138]. Fever, elevated ESR, neutrophilia, and polyclonal gammopathy are other common associations.

3.3.6 Xanthoma disseminatum

It occurs in children and adults and characterized by disseminated xanthomatous lesions. XD usually presents as erythematous, yellow brown papule and nodules, symmetrical in distribution. Lesions become confluent, sometimes form a xanthomatous plaque, and may become verrucous [139].

It usually starts before the age of 25 years in about 60% of patients. It is more common in males. It may occur anywhere on the body including the scalp, face, trunk, and extremities [140].

XD typically involves the skin, particularly the flexor folds, face, and trunk. It may also manifest in the central nervous system [141].

Mucous membrane involvement develops in 40–60% of patients, most commonly affecting the oropharynx, larynx, or cornea and conjunctiva [142].

There are three clinical patterns of xanthoma disseminatum: (i) a common persistent form in which lesions may never resolve; (ii) a rare, self-healing form with spontaneous resolution; and (iii) a very rare, progressive form with organ dysfunction and central nervous system involvement [143].

3.4 Other granulomatous disorders

3.4.1 Granulomatous vasculitis

Granulomatous vasculitis is a spectrum of diseases. Lung involvement is very much common in GV. Small vessel vasculitis with granulomatosis is seen in granulomatosis with polyangiitis (Wegener granulomatosis) and eosinophilic granulomatosis with polyangiitis (Churg-Strauss syndrome), and large-vessel vasculitis with granulomatosis is seen in temporal arteritis: Takayasu arteritis.

In Wegener granulomatosis, the incidence of skin disease is 45% [144]. The lesions can take several forms including papules, vesicles, palpable purpura, ulcers, and subcutaneous nodules [145]. Palpable purpura may be the most frequent (47%) skin finding [146]. The skin disease rarely dominates the clinical picture and is usually a minor part of the multisystem involvement, generally responds promptly to therapy, and parallels disease activity in other organ systems [147]. Other organs include the lungs, kidney, heart, joint, eye, and nervous system involvement [148]. Cutaneous findings are variable and nonspecific and usually affect the lower extremities [146].

Eosinophilic granulomatosis with polyangiitis was previously named as Churg-Strauss syndrome. In one-third to two-thirds of patients, skin involvement is a dominant feature and presents in the form of nodules. Urticaria and ulceration are less common. Neurologic involvement is seen in 60–70% patients and is commonly in the form of multiple mononeuropathies or symmetric polyneuropathy [149].

3.4.2 Lymphomatoid granulomatosis

Lymphomatoid granulomatosis (LYG) is a progressive lymphoproliferative disease by Epstein-Barr virus (EBV), in which the abnormal cells directly accumulate within affected tissues, usually in the form of infiltrative nodular lesions and with T-cell invasion and destruction of blood vessels [150]. Its incidence is low, clinical features are overlapping, pulmonary disorders are more common, and all contribute to frequent delays in diagnosis [150]. The lung is virtually always involved in bilateral fashion [151]. The skin is the extrapulmonary organ most commonly involved in LYG, occurring in 40–50% of patients [151]. Skin manifestations of LYG are quite heterogeneous. They typically appear as scattered subcutaneous or dermal nodules that vary in size, seen predominantly on the extremities. Erythematous or purplish maculopapular eruptions are the most common skin lesions observed, but some patients will have indurated plaques. Varying degrees of ulceration accompany the skin lesions and may become necrotic when the disease is not well controlled (**Figure 23**). In up to 10% of patients, the skin lesions will antedate the lung lesions, and, in these cases, dermal biopsy may lead to the diagnosis [150]. Skin lesion may develop after lung involvement, but majority of skin lesions develop at the time of lung involvement [151].

3.4.3 Foreign body reactions

The foreign body granuloma is a response of biological tissue to any foreign material in the tissue [152]. Foreign body granulomas may be due to reactions of endogenous products like keratin, hair, fat, urate crystals, mineral, and/or oil products; plant and animal products; and synthetic agents [153]. Depending on the individual host response and type of foreign materials, clinical findings can be variable. Sites depend on the area involved by endo- or exogenous material. The lesions may be asymptomatic or tender, pink, red, red-brown or skin-colored, and firm papules, nodules, or plaques, which may or may not ulcerate or drain (**Figure 24**). Other presentations include sinus tracts and abscesses [153]. The foreign material may migrate, as in silicone, leading to granulomas at sites distant from the area of implantation [154].

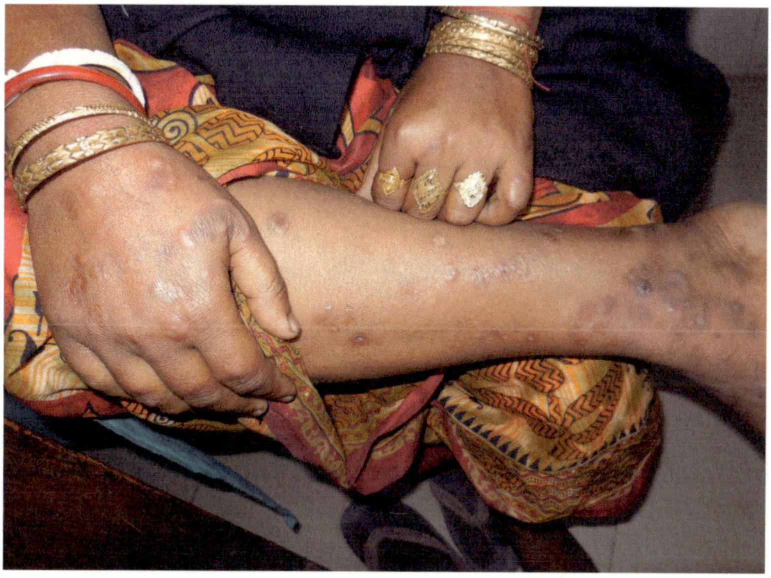

Figure 23.
Lymphomatoid granulomatosis.

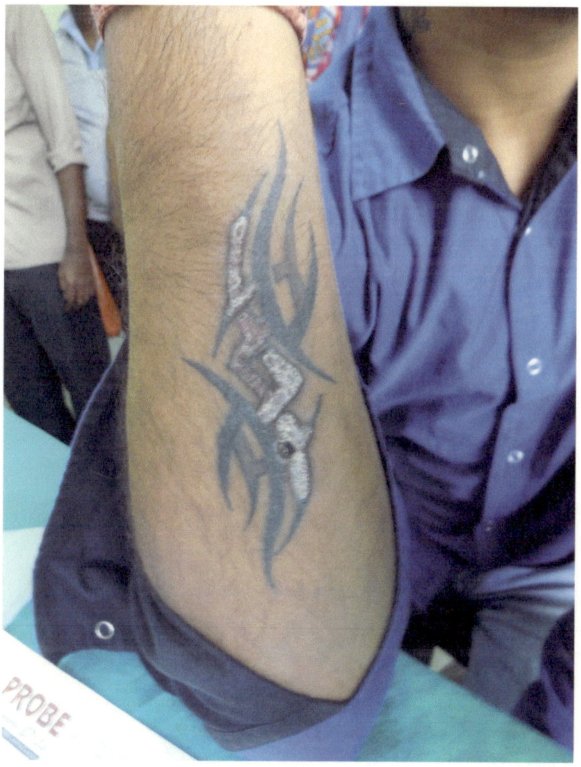

Figure 24.
Foreign body granuloma.

3.4.4 Granulomatous drug reactions

Granulomatous drug reactions include four major types: interstitial granulomatous drug reaction, drug-induced accelerated rheumatoid nodulosis, drug-induced granuloma annulare, and drug-induced sarcoidosis [155].

The most common cutaneous features of interstitial granulomatous drug reaction are symptomatic erythematous plaques and papules with a predilection for the flexures (intertriginous areas, medial thighs, and inner aspects of the arms) [117]. Trunks also may be involved [117]. Sharply demarcated symmetrical annular erythematous lesions [155] are also described. Lesions may be generalized [117]. Interstitial granulomatous drug reaction completely regresses with drug cessation [155]. Other drug-induced granulomatous disorders are drug-induced accelerated rheumatoid nodulosis, with development of tender subcutaneous lesions during treatment with methotrexate, and drug-induced granuloma annulare (GA), mainly generalized, developed with paroxetine and drug-induced sarcoidosis [156]. Drug-induced lesions are similar to the original lesions.

Author details

Suchibrata Das
Department of Dermatology, Venereology and Leprosy, Nilratan Sircar Medical College, West Bengal, India

*Address all correspondence to: suchibratadas@yahoo.com

References

[1] Geraint James D. A clinicopathological classification of granulomatous disorders. Postgraduate Medical Journal. 2000;**76**:457-465

[2] Lapointe A-K, Laffitte E. Disseminated cutaneous granulomatosis. Revue Médicale Suisse. 2009;**5**(900):902-906

[3] Asai J. What is new in the histogenesis of granulomatous skin diseases? The Journal of Dermatology. 2017;**44**(3): 297-303. DOI: 10.1111/1346-8138.13662

[4] English JC, Rosenbach M. F092—Granulomatous disorders of adult skin. In: 76th Annual Meeting San Diego, CA USA. American Academy of Dermatology. 2018. Available from: www.aad.org.faculty.handout

[5] Sanchez M, Prystowsky S. Sarcoidosis of the skin. In: Basow D, editor. UpToDate. Waltham, MA: UpToDate; 2010

[6] Sam WM, Lynch PJ, editors. Principles and Practice of Dermatology. 2nd ed. New York: Churchill Livingstone; 1996. pp. 629-639

[7] Elgart ML. Cutaneous sarcoidosis: Definitions and types of lesions. Clinics in Dermatology. 1986;**4**:35-45

[8] Gawkrodger DJ. Sarcoidosis. In: Burns T, Breathnach S, Cox N, Griffiths C, editors. Rook's Textbook of Dermatology. 8th ed. Oxford: Wiley-Blackwell; 2010. pp. 61.1-61.23

[9] Scadding JG, Mitchell DN, editors. Sarcoidosis of the Skin. London: Chapman & Hall Medical; 1985. pp. 181-206

[10] Mañá J, Marcoval J, Graells J, Salazar A, Peyrí J, Pujol R. Cutaneous involvement in sarcoidosis. Relationship to systemic disease. Archives of Dermatology. 1997;**133**:882-888

[11] James DG. Dermatological aspects of sarcoidosis. The Quarterly Journal of Medicine. 1959;**28**:109-124

[12] Veien NK, Stahl D, Brodthagen H. Cutaneous sarcoidosis in Caucasians. Journal of the American Academy of Dermatology. 1987;**16**:534-540

[13] Sharma OP. Cutaneous sarcoidosis: Clinical features and management. Chest. 1972;**61**:320-325

[14] Marcoval J, Mana J. Sarcoidosis. In: Girffiths C, Barker J, Bleiker T, Chalmers R, Creamer D, editors. Rook's Textbook of Dermatology. 9th ed. West Sussex, UK; 2016. pp. 98.1-98.17

[15] Jorizzo JL, Koufman JA, Thompson JN, White WL, Shar GG, Schreiner DJ. Sarcoidosis of the upper respiratory tract in patients with nasal rim lesions: A pilot study. Journal of the American Academy of Dermatology. 1990;**22**:439-443

[16] Kerdel FA, Moschella SL. Sarcoidosis: An updated review. Journal of the American Academy of Dermatology. 1984;**11**:1-19

[17] Callen JP. Relationship of cutaneous sarcoidosis to systemic disease. Clinics in Dermatology. 1986:446-453

[18] Moschella SL. Disease of the mononuclear phagocytic system. In: Moschella SL, Hurley HJ, editors. Dermatology. Philadelphia: WB Saunders; 1985. pp. 915-916

[19] Scheig RL. Sarcoidosis. In: Demis DJ, editor. Clinical Dermatology. Philadelphia: JB Lippincott; 1988. pp. 1-5

[20] English JC III, Patel PJ, Greer KE. Sarcoidosis. Journal of the American Academy of Dermatology. 2001;**44**:725-743

[21] Spiteri MA, Matthey F, Gordon T, et al. Lupus pernio. A clinico-radiological study of thirty-five cases. The British Journal of Dermatology. 1985;**112**:315-322

[22] Paller AS, Surek C, Silva-Walsh I, Krespi Y, Freinkel RK. Cutaneous sarcoidosis associated with sarcoidosis of the upper airway. Archives of Dermatology. 1983;**119**:592-596

[23] Neville E, Mills RG, James DG. Sarcoidosis of the upper respiratory tract and its relation to lupus pernio. Annals of the New York Academy of Sciences. 1976;**278**:416-426

[24] James DG. Lupus pernio. Lupus. 1992;**1**:129-131

[25] Young RJ 3rd, Gilson RT, Yanase D, Elston DM. Cutaneous sarcoidosis. International Journal of Dermatology. 2001;**40**:249-253

[26] Henrichs MP, Streitbürger A, Gosheger G, Surke C, Dierkes C, Hardes J. Scar sarcoidosis on a finger mimicking a rapidly growing soft tissue tumour: A case report. BMC Research Notes. 2012;**5**:545-549. DOI: 10.1186/1756-0500-5-545

[27] Choi SY, Hyun MY, No YA, Park KY, Li K, Kim BJ, et al. Scar sarcoidosis on a hypertrophic scar. Clinical and Experimental Dermatology. 2014;**39**:945-947. DOI: 10.1111/ced.12417

[28] Cervigon I, Palomo A, Torres LM. Cutaneous lesions on scars. Actas Dermo-Sifiliográficas. 2007;**98**:433-434 (in Spanish)

[29] Marchell RM, Judson MA. Chronic cutaneous lesions of sarcoidosis. Clinics in Dermatology. 2007;**25**:295-302. DOI: 10.1016/j.clindermatol.2007.03.007

[30] Marcoval J, Mañá J, Rubio M. Specific cutaneous lesions in patients with systemic sarcoidosis: Relationship to severity and chronicity of disease. Clinical and Experimental Dermatology. 2011;**36**:739-744. DOI: 10.1111/j.1365-2230.2011.04128.x

[31] Ahmed I, Harshad SR. Subcutaneous sarcoidosis: Is it a specific subset of cutaneous sarcoidosis frequently associated with systemic disease? Journal of the American Academy of Dermatology. 2006;**54**(1):p55-p60

[32] Mahajan VK, Sharma NL, Sharma RC, Sharma VC. Cutaneous sarcoidosis: Clinical profile of 23 Indian patients. Indian Journal of Dermatology, Venereology and Leprology. 2007;**73**: 16-21

[33] James WD, Berger TG, Elston DM, editors. Macrophage/monocyte disorders. In: Andrews' Diseases of the Skin. 12th ed. Philadelphia: Elsevier; 2016. pp. 699-725

[34] Arias Santiago S, Fernández-Pugnaire MA, Aneiros-Fernández J, Falcón CS, Callejas-Rubio JL, Ortego-Centeno N, et al. Recurrent telangiectasias on the cheek: Angiolupoid sarcoidosis. The American Journal of Medicine. 2010;**123**(1):e7-e8. DOI: 10.1016/j.amjmed.2009.08.014

[35] Meyrick RH, Thomas MA, McKee PH, Black MM. Hypopigmented sarcoidosis. Journal of the Royal Society of Medicine. 1981;**74**

[36] Clayton R, Breathnach A, Martin B, Feiwel M. Hypopigmented sarcoidosis in the negro report of eight cases with ultrastructural observations. British Journal of Dermatology. 1977;**96**:119

[37] Burov EA, Kantor GR, Isaac M. Morpheaform sarcoidosis: Report of three cases. Journal of the American Academy of Dermatology. 1998;**39**(2):345-348. DOI: 10.1016/s0190-9622(98)70386-x

[38] Choi S-C, Kim H-J, Kim C-R, Byun J-Y, Lee D-Y, Lee J-H, et al. A case of morpheaform sarcoidosis. Annals of Dermatology. 2010;**22**(3):316-318

[39] Klauder JV. Multiple sarcoid-like granulomas of the skin. Archiv für Dermatologie und Syphilis. 1925;**12**:171-173

[40] Elgart ML. Skin manifestations of sarcoidosis. Cutis. 1968;**1**:283-291

[41] Fujii K, Okamoto H, Onuki M, et al. Recurrent follicular and lichenoid papules of sarcoidosis. Europcan Journal of Dermatology. 2000;**10**:303-305

[42] Seo SK, Yeum JS, Suh JC, Na GY. Lichenoid sarcoidosis in a 3-year-old girl. Pediatric Dermatology. 2001;**18**:384-387

[43] Sinha P, Bhattacharjee S, Raman DK, Sood A. A rare case of lichenoid sarcoidosis mimicking papular amyloidosis. Indian Journal of Dermatology. 2020;**65**:50-52

[44] Vazquez-Lopez F, Palacios-Garcia L, Gomez-Diez S, Argenziano G. Dermoscopy for discriminating between lichenoid sarcoidosis and lichen planus. Archives of Dermatology. 2011;**147**:1130

[45] Albertini JG. Ulcerative sarcoidosis. Archives of Dermatology. 1997;**133**(2):215. DOI: 10.1001/archderm.1997.03890380087013

[46] Verdegem TD, Sharma OP. Cutaneous ulcers in sarcoidosis. Archives of Dermatology. 1987;**123**:1531-1534

[47] Shmunes E. Verrucose sarcoidosis. Archives of Dermatology. 1970;**102**(6):665. DOI: 10.1001/archderm.1970.04000120083016

[48] Stockman DL, Rosenberg J, Bengana C, Suster S, Plaza JA. Verrucous cutaneous sarcoidosis. The American Journal of Dermatopathology. 2013;**35**(2):273-276. DOI: 10.1097/dad.0b013e318262ed4c

[49] James DG, Neville E, Siltzbach LE. A worldwide review of sarcoidosis. Annals of the New York Academy of Sciences. 1976;**278**:321-334

[50] Chowaniec M, Starba A, Wiland P. Erythema nodosum—Review of the literature. Reumatologia. 2016;**54**(2):79-82

[51] Milman N, Selroos O. Pulmonary sarcoidosis in the Nordic countries 1950-1982. Epidemiology and clinical picture. Sarcoidosis. 1990;**7**:50-57

[52] Sö derstrom RM, Krull EA. Erythema nodosum: A review. Cutis. 1978;**21**:806-810

[53] Requena L, Yus ES. Erythema nodosum. Dermatologic Clinics. 2008;**26**(4):425-438. DOI: 10.1016/j.det.2008.05.014

[54] Blake T, Manahan M, Rodins K. Erythema nodosum—A review of an uncommon panniculitis. Dermatology Online Journal. 2014;**20**(4):22376

[55] Psychos DN, Voulgari PV, Skopouli FN, et al. Erythema nodosum: The underlying conditions. Clinical Rheumatology. 2000;**19**:212-216

[56] Kakourou T, Drosatou P, Psychou F, et al. Erythema nodosum in children. Journal of the American Academy of Dermatology. 2001;**44**:17-21

[57] Gran JT, Bohmer E. Acute sarcoid arthritis: A favourable outcome? A retrospective survey of 49 patients with review of the literature. Scandinavian Journal of Rheumatology. 1996;**25**:70-73

[58] Kang EH. Sarcoidosis in Korea: Revisited. Journal of the Korean Medical Association. 2008;**51**:925-932

[59] Zisman DA, Shorr AF, Lynch JP 3rd. Sarcoidosis involving the musculoskeletal system. Seminars in Respiratory and Critical Care Medicine. 2002;**23**:555-570

[60] Mana J, Gormez-Vaquero C, Montero A, Salazar A, Marcoval J, Valverde J, et al. Lofgren's syndrome revisited: A study of 186 patients. The American Journal of Medicine. 1999;**107**:240-245

[61] James DG, Neville E, Carstairs LS. Bone and joint sarcoidosis. Seminars in Arthritis and Rheumatism. 1976;**6**:53-81

[62] Lofgren S, Lundback H. The bilateral hilar lymphoma syndrome; a study of the relation to tuberculosis and sarcoidosis in 212 cases. Acta Medica Scandinavica. 1952;**142**:265-273

[63] Lewandowsky F. Uber Rosacea-ahnliche Tuberkulide des Geschites. Corr BI Schweiz Arzte. 1917;**47**:1280-1282

[64] van Ketel WG. Rosacea-like tuberculid of Lewandowsky. Dermatologica. 1958;**116**:201-210

[65] Mullanax MG, Kierland RR. Granulomatous rosacea. Archives of Dermatology. 1970;**101**:206-211

[66] Wilkin J, Dahl M, Detmar M, et al. Standard classification of rosacea: Report of the National Rosacea Society Expert Committee on the classification and staging of rosacea. Journal of the American Academy of Dermatology. 2002;**46**:584-587

[67] Crawford GH, Pelle MT, James WD. Rosacea: I. Etiology, pathogenesis, and subtype classification. Journal of the American Academy of Dermatology. 2004;**51**:327-341

[68] Wilkin J, Dahl M, Detmar M, et al. Standard grading system for rosacea: Report of the National Rosacea Society Expert Committee on the classification and staging of rosacea. Journal of the American Academy of Dermatology. 2004;**50**:907-912

[69] Khokhar O, Khachemoune A. A case of granulomatous rosacea: Sorting granulomatous rosacea from other granulomatous diseases that affect the face. Dermatology Online Journal. 2004;**10**:6

[70] Helm KF, Menz J, Gibson LE, et al. A clinical and histopathologic study of granulomatous rosacea. Journal of the American Academy of Dermatology. 1991;**25**(6 pt 1):1038-1043

[71] Sánchez JL, Berlingeri-Ramos AC, Dianette Vázquez D. Granulomatous rosacea. The American Journal of Dermatopathology. 2008;**30**:6-9

[72] Danese S, Semeraro S, Papa A, et al. Extraintestinal manifestations in inflammatory bowel disease. World Journal of Gastroenterology. 2005;**11**:7227-7236

[73] Kurtzman DJ, Jones T, Lian F, Peng LS. Metastatic Crohn's disease: A review and approach to therapy. Journal of the American Academy of Dermatology. DOI: 10.1016/j.jaad.2014.04.002

[74] Crowson AN, Nuovo GJ, Mihm MC Jr, Magro C. Cutaneous manifestations of Crohn's disease, its spectrum and its pathogenesis: Intracellular consensus bacterial 16S rRNA is associated with the gastrointestinal but not the cutaneous manifestations of Crohn's disease. Human Pathology. 2003;**34**:1185-1192

[75] Albuquerque A, Magro F, Rodrigues S, Lopes J, Lopes S, Dias JM, et al. Metastatic cutaneous Crohn's disease of the face: A case report and review of the literature. European Journal of Gastroenterology & Hepatology. 2011;**23**:954-956

[76] Chen W, Blume-Peytavi U, Goerdt S, Orfanos CE. Metastatic Crohn's disease of the face. Journal of the American Academy of Dermatology. 1996;**35**:986-988

[77] Palamaras I, El-Jabbour J, Pietropaolo N, Thomson P, Mann S, Robles W, et al. Metastatic Crohn's disease: A review. Journal of the European Academy of Dermatology and Venereology. 2008;**22**:1033-1043

[78] Issa MA. Crohn's disease of the mouth. British Dental Journal. 1971;**130**:247-248

[79] Wiesenfeld D, Ferguson MM, Mitchell DN, et al. Orofacial granulomatosis—A clinical and pathological analysis. The Quarterly Journal of Medicine. 1985;**54**:101-113

[80] Mignogna MD, Fedele S, Lo Russo L, Lo Muzio L. The multiform and variable patterns of onset of orofacial granulomatosis. Journal of Oral Pathology & Medicine. 2003;**32**:200-205

[81] Grave B, McCullough M, Wiesenfeld D. Orofacial granulomatosis—A 20-year review. Oral Diseases. 2009;**15**(1):46-51. DOI: 10.1111/j.1601-0825.2008.01500.x

[82] Singhal P, Chandan GD, Das UM, Singhal A. A rare case report of orofacial granulomatosis in a pediatric patient. Journal of the Indian Society of Pedodontics and Preventive Dentistry. 2012;**30**:262-266

[83] Piette EW, Rosenbach M. Granuloma annulare. Clinical and histologic variants, epidemiology, and genetics. Journal of the American Academy of Dermatology. 2016;**75**:457-465

[84] Muhlbauer JE. Granuloma annulare. Journal of the American Academy of Dermatology. 1980;**3**:217-230

[85] Cyr PR. Diagnosis and management of granuloma annulare. American Family Physician. 2006;**74**:1729-1734

[86] Dabski K, Winkelmann RK. Generalized granuloma annulare: Histopathology and immunopathology. Systematic review of 100 cases and comparison with localized granuloma annulare. Journal of the American Academy of Dermatology. 1989;**20**:28-39

[87] McDermott MB, Lind AC, Marley EF, et al. Deep granuloma annulare (pseudorheumatoid nodule) in children: Clinicopathologic study of 35 cases. Pediatric and Developmental Pathology. 1998;**1**:300-308

[88] Felner EI, Steinberg JB, Weinberg AG. Subcutaneous granuloma annulare: A review of 47 cases. Pediatrics. 1997;**100**:965-967

[89] De Aloe G, Risulo M, Sbano P, Pianigiani E, Fimiani M. Congenital subcutaneous granuloma annulare. Pediatric Dermatology. 2005;**22**(3):234-236. DOI: 10.1111/j.1525-1470.2005.22311.x

[90] Goncalves RR et al. Annular elastolytic giant cell granuloma—Case report. Anais Brasileiros de Dermatologia. 2011;**86**:S69-S71

[91] Arora S, Malik A, Patil C, Balki A. Annular elastolytic giant cell granuloma: A report of 10 cases. Indian Dermatology Online Journal. 2015;**6**(Suppl S1):17-20

[92] Ishibashi A, Yokoyama A, Hirano K. Annular elastolytic giant cell granuloma occurring in covered areas. Dermatologica. 1987;**174**:293

[93] Kato H et al. Annular elastolytic giant cell granuloma: An unusual case with papular lesions. The Journal of Dermatology. 1991;**18**:667

[94] Meadows KP, O'Reilly MA, Harris RM, Petersen MJ. Erythematous annular plaques in a necklace distribution. Archives of Dermatology. 2001;**137**:1647-1652

[95] Gutierrez-Gonzalez E, Gomez-Bernal S, Alvarez-Perez A, Sanchez-Aguilar D, Toribio J. Elastolytic giant cell granuloma: Clinic-pathologic review of twenty cases. Dermatology Online Journal. 2013;**19**:20019

[96] Shoimer I, Wismer J. Annular elastolytic giant cell granuloma associated with temporal arteritis leading to blindness. Journal of Cutaneous Medicine and Surgery. 2011;**15**(5):293-297

[97] Djilali-Bouzina F, Grange F, Krzisch S, Schnebelen MP, Grosshans E, Guillaume JC. Annular elastolytic giant cell granuloma. Annales de Dermatologie et de Vénéréologie. 2010;**137**(8-9):536-540

[98] Rongioletti F, Baldari M, Burlando M, Parodi A. Papular elastolytic giant cell granuloma: Report of a case associated with monoclonal gammopathy and responsive to topical tacrolimus. Clinical and Experimental Dermatology. 2010;**35**(2):145-148

[99] Das S, Chowdhury J, Patra S, Achar A. Annular elastolytic giant cell granuloma—A rare case with systemic involvement. Bangladesh Journal of Medical Science. 2016;**15**:488-491

[100] Muller SA, Winkelmann RK. Necrobiosis lipoidica diabetico-rum: A clinical and pathological investigation of 171 cases. Archives of Dermatology. 1966;**93**:272-281

[101] Peyri J, Moreno A, Marcoval J. Necrobiosis lipoidica. Seminars in Cutaneous Medicine and Surgery. 2007;**26**:87-89

[102] Reid SD, Ladizinski B, Lee K, Baibergenova A, Alavi A. Update on necrobiosis lipoidica: A review of etiology, diagnosis, and treatment options. Journal of the American Academy of Dermatology. 2013;**69**:783-791

[103] Thomas M, Khopkar US. Necrobiosis lipoidica: A clinicopathological study in the Indian scenario. Indian Dermatology Online Journal. 2013;**4**:288-291

[104] Mann RJ, Harman RRM. Cutaneous anaesthesia in necrobiosis lipoidica. British Journal of Dermatology. 1984;**110**(3):323-325. DOI: 10.1111/j.1365-2133.1984

[105] Santos-Juanes J, Galache C, Curto JR, Carrasco MP, Ribas A, Sanchez del Rio J. Squamous cell carcinoma arising in long-standing necrobiosis lipoidica. Journal of the European Academy of Dermatology and Venereology. 2004;**18**:199-200

[106] Sayah A, English JC 3rd. Rheumatoid arthritis: A review of the cutaneous manifestations. Journal of the American Academy of Dermatology. 2005;**53**(2):191-209 quiz 210-2

[107] Ziff M. The rheumatoid nodule. Arthritis and Rheumatism. 1990;**33**(6):761-767. DOI: 10.1002/art.1780330601

[108] Gordon DA, Stein JL, Broder I. The extra-articular features of rheumatoid arthritis. A systematic analysis of 127 cases. The American Journal of Medicine. 1973;**54**:445-452

[109] Wood MG, Beerman H. Necrobiosis lipoidica granuloma annulare and rheumatoid nodule. Journal of Investigative Dermatology. 1960;**34**:139-147

[110] Kaye BR, Kaye RL, Bobrove A. Rheumatoid nodules. Review of the spectrum of associated conditions and proposal of a new classification, with

a report of four seronegative cases. The American Journal of Medicine. 1984;**76**:279-292

[111] Rosenbach M, English JC 3rd. Reactive granulomatous dermatitis: A review of palisaded neutrophilic and granulomatous dermatitis, interstitial granulomatous dermatitis, interstitial granulomatous drug reaction, and a proposed reclassification. Dermatologic Clinics. 2015;**33**(3):373-387

[112] Chu P, Connolly MK, LeBoit PE. The histopathologic spectrum of palisaded neutrophilic and granulomatous dermatitis in patients with collagen vascular disease. Archives of Dermatology. 1994;**130**:1278-1283

[113] Finan MC, Winkelmann RK. The cutaneous extravascular necrotizing granuloma (Churg-Strauss granuloma) and systemic disease: A review of 27 cases. Medicine (Baltimore). 1983;**62**:142-158

[114] Hantash BM, Chiang D, Kohler S, et al. Palisaded neutrophilic and granulomatous dermatitis associated with limited systemic sclerosis. Journal of the American Academy of Dermatology. 2008;**58**:661-664

[115] Dykman CJ, Galens GJ, Good AE. Linear subcutaneous bands in rheumatoid arthritis. Annals of Internal Medicine. 1965;**63**:134-140

[116] Peroni A, Colato C, Schena D, et al. Interstitial granulomatous dermatitis: A distinct entity with characteristic histological and clinical pattern. The British Journal of Dermatology. 2011;**166**:775-783

[117] Magro CM, Crowson AN, Schapiro BL. The interstitial granulomatous drug reaction: A distinctive clinical and pathological entity. Journal of Cutaneous Pathology. 1998;**25**:72-78

[118] Luz FB, Gaspar AP, Kalil-Gaspar N, Ramos-e-Silva M. Histiocytes and non-Langerhans cell histiocytoses in dermatology. Anais Brasileiros de Dermatologia. 2003;**78**:99-118

[119] Achar A, Naskar B, Mondal PC, Pal M. Multiple generalized xanthogranuloma in adult: Case report and treatment. Indian Journal of Dermatology. 2011;**56**:197-199

[120] Chisolm SS, Schulman JM, Fox LP. Adult xanthogranuloma, reticulohistiocytosis, and Rosai-Dorfman disease. Dermatologic Clinics. 2015;**33**:465-472

[121] Saad N, Skowron F, Dalle S, Forestier JY, Balme B, Thomas L. Multiple adult xanthogranuloma: Case report and literature review. Dermatology. 2006;**212**:73-76

[122] Caputo R, Grimalt R, Gelmetti C, Cottoni F. Unusual aspects of juvenile xanthogranuloma. Journal of the American Academy of Dermatology. 1993;**29**:868-870

[123] Jakobiec FA, Mills MD, Hidayat AA, et al. Periocular xanthogranulomas associated with severe adult-onset asthma. Transactions of the American Ophthalmological Society. 1993;**91**:99-125

[124] Sivak-Callcott JA, Rootman J, Rasmussen SL, et al. Adult xanthogranulomatous disease of the orbit and ocular adnexa: New immunohistochemical findings and clinical review. The British Journal of Ophthalmology. 2006;**90**:602-608

[125] London J, Martin A, Soussan M, Badelon I, Gille T, Uzunhan Y, et al. Adult onset asthma and periocular xanthogranuloma (AAPOX), a rare entity with a strong link to IgG4-related disease. Medicine (Baltimore). 2015;**94**(43):e1916

[126] Nelson CA, Zhong CS, Hashemi DA, Ashchyan HJ, Brown-Joel Z, Noe MH, et al. A multicenter cross-sectional study and systematic review of necrobiotic xanthogranuloma with proposed diagnostic criteria. JAMA Dermatology. 2020. DOI: 10.1001/jamadermatol.2019.4221

[127] Mehregan DA, Winkelmann RK. Necrobiotic xanthogranuloma. Archives of Dermatology. 1992;**128**:94-100

[128] Girisha BS, Holla AP, Fernandes M, Noronha TM. Necrobiotic xanthogranuloma. Journal of Cutaneous and Aesthetic Surgery. 2012;**5**(1):43-45

[129] Rao AG, Lakshmi TS, Vani V. Multicentric reticulohistiocytosis. Indian Journal of Dermatology, Venereology and Leprology. 2003;**69**:35-36

[130] Trotta F, Castellino G, Monaco AL. Multicentric reticulohistiocytosis. Best Practice & Research. Clinical Rheumatology. 2004;**5**:759-772

[131] Barrow MV, Holubar K. Multicentric reticulohistiocytosis. A review of 33 patients. Medicine (Baltimore). 1969;**48**:287-305

[132] Rapini RP. Multicentric reticulohistiocytosis. Clinics in Dermatology. 1993;**11**:107-111

[133] Luz FB, Gaspar NK, Gaspar AP, Carneiro S, Ramos-e-Silva M. Multicentric reticulohistiocytosis: A proliferation of macrophages with tropism for skin and joints, part I. Skinmed. 2007;**6**:172-178

[134] Sinha A, Dhungana S, Dipankar D, Prakash M, Sharma SK, Das A. Multicentric reticulohistiocytosis: A clinicoradiological review. Indian Journal of Rheumatology. 2018;**13**:195-201

[135] Farraj S. Familial histiocytic dermatoarthritis. A new syndrome. American Journal of Medicine. 1973;**54**:793-800

[136] Pennys NS, Ahn YS, McKinney EC, McCleod T, Byrne G Jr, Byrnes J, et al. Sinus histiocytosis with massive lymphadenopathy. A case with unusual skin involvement and a therapeutic response to vinblastine loaded platelets. Cancer. 1982;**49**:1994-1998

[137] Innocenzi D, Silipo V, Giombini S, Ruco L, Bosman C, Calviero S. Sinus histiocytes with massive lymphadenopathy-Rosai-Dorfman syndrome: Case report with nodal and diffuse mucocutaneous involvement. Journal of Cutaneous Pathology. 1998;**25**:563-567

[138] Sanchez R, Rosai J, Dorfman RF. Sinus histiocytosis with massive lymphadenopathy. An analysis of 113 cases with special emphasis on its extranodal manifestations. Laboratory Investigation. 1977;**36**:21-22

[139] Tran TH, Pope E, Weitzman S. Cutaneous histiocytosis. In: Griffiths C, Barker J, Bleiker J, Chelmers R, Creamer D, editors. Rooks Textbook of Dermatology. 9th ed

[140] Kang TW, Kim SC. A case of xanthoma disseminatum presenting as pedunculating nodules and plaques. Korean Journal of Dermatology. 2007;**45**:290-293

[141] Alexander AS, Turner R, Uniate L, Pearcy RG. Xanthoma disseminatum: A case report and literature review. The British Journal of Radiology. 2005;**78**:153-157

[142] Rupec RA, Schaller M. Xanthoma disseminatum. International Journal of Dermatology. 2002;**41**:911-913

[143] Seaton ED, Pillai GJ, Chu AC. Treatment of xanthoma disseminatum with cyclophosphamide. The British Journal of Dermatology. 2004;**150**:346-349

[144] Wolff SM. Wegener's granulomatosis. Annals of Internal Medicine. 1974;**81**(4):513. DOI: 10.7326/0003-4819-81-4-513

[145] Fauci AS, Wolff SM. Wegener's granulomatosis: Studies in eighteen patients and a review of the literature. Medicine (Baltimore). 1973;**52**:535-561

[146] Daoud MS, Gibson LE, DeRemee RA, Specks U, El-Azhary RA, Daniel Su WP. Cutaneous Wegener's granulomatosis: Clinical, histopathologic, and immunopathologic features of thirty patients. Journal of the American Academy of Dermatology. 1994;**31**(4):605-612. DOI: 10.1016/s0190-9622(94)70224-1

[147] Fauci AS, Haynes BF, Katz P. The spectrum of vasculitis: Clinical, pathologic, immunologic, and therapeutic considerations. Annals of Internal Medicine. 1978;**89**:660-676

[148] Fauci AS. Wegener's granulomatosis: Prospective clinical and therapeutic experience with 85 patients for 21 years. Annals of Internal Medicine. 1983;**98**(1):76. DOI: 10.7326/0003-4819-98-1-76.

[149] Sharma A, Dogra S, Sharma K. Granulomatous vasculitis. Dermatologic Clinics. 2015;**33**:475-487

[150] Roschewski M, Wilson WH. Lymphomatoid granulomatosis. The Cancer Journal. 2012;**18**(5):469-474. DOI: 10.1097/ppo.0b013e31826c5e19

[151] Katzenstein AL, Carrington CB, Liebow AA. Lymphomatoid granulomatosis: A clinicopathologic study of 152 cases. Cancer. 1979;**43**:360-373

[152] Rapini RP, Bolognia JL, Jorizzo JL. Dermatology: 2-Volume Set. St. Louis: Mosby; 2007. p. 1443. ISBN: 978-1-4160-2999-1

[153] Hirsch BC, Johnson WC. Pathology of granulomatous diseases: Foreign body granulomas. International Journal of Dermatology. 1984;**23**:531-538

[154] Delage C, Shane JJ, Johnson FB. Mammary silicone granuloma: Migration of silicone fluid to abdominal wall and inguinal region. Archives of Dermatology. 1973;**108**:104-107

[155] Dodiuk-Gad RP, Shear NH. Granulomatous drug eruptions. Dermatologic Clinics. 2015;**33**:525-539

[156] Laura A, Luca P, Luisa PA. Interstitial granulomatous drug reaction due to febuxostat. Indian Journal of Dermatology, Venereology and Leprology. 2014;**80**(2):182-184

Chapter 6

Granulomatous Interstitial Nephritis in Children Resulting from Wegener's Granulomatosis, Crohn's Disease, or Sarcoidosis

Galina Makovetskaya, Lilia Mazur and Elena Balashova

Abstract

Granulomatous interstitial nephritis (GIN) is a rare type of kidney disease, the precise etiology of which is obscure, but is most commonly seen following drug therapy and infection. The main infections seen in the onset of this pathology, especially in immunocompromised patients, include mycobacteria and fungi. Granulomatous interstitial nephritis can be a manifestation of systemic diseases, such as Wegener's granulomatosis, Crohn's disease, or sarcoidosis. We present our experience with GIN diagnosis and management.

Keywords: granulomatous interstitial nephritis, chronic kidney disease, children, toxocariasis, chronic granulomatous disease

1. Introduction

Granulomatous inflammation is a chronic inflammatory reaction, the main feature of which is the cellular transformation of a monocyte into a macrophage—a multinucleate giant epithelioid cell. The most common cause of this transformation is incomplete phagocytosis.

Difficulties in the clinical diagnosis of granulomatous interstitial nephritis (GIN) relate to the lack of a reliable noninvasive diagnostic method. Granulomatous interstitial nephritis is a rare type of kidney disease with a frequency of no more than 1%, according to the data at hand [1]. The precise cause of GIN is not known; due to the rarity of the disease, researchers rely primarily on a series of cases, rather than on the results of multicenter studies. In addition, the etiological structure of GIN can vary in different countries: in more developed countries, GIN is more probably related to drugs and sarcoidosis, whereas in less developed regions, it is likely to be associated with infections [2]. However, the most common causes are drug therapy and infection, and drugs (NSAIDs, antimicrobials, anticonvulsants, diuretics, and allopurinol) [3–5] account for 9–45% [6, 7] up to 55–70% [1], according to different studies.

The main infectious factors in the onset of this pathology, especially in immunocompromised patients, include mycobacteria [7] and fungi [1, 7]. GIN can be associated with HIV infection [8] and the influenza A (H1N1) virus [9]. Patients with GIN of infectious etiology were stated to have acute kidney damage at onset [6]. In some cases, the etiology of GIN cannot be pinpointed; thus, the disease is considered to be idiopathic [3, 10]. GIN resulting in nephrosclerosis and chronic pathology of the digestive organs, and atopic dermatitis associated with carriage of *Toxocara*, has been reported.

We had a patient born with a body weight of 2.0 kg after an uneventful first pregnancy whose infantile period was unremarkable. When the girl was 1.5 years old, she suffered a common form of atopic dermatitis with periodic exacerbations (treated with topical steroids during exacerbations). At the age of 3 years, she was seen by a gastroenterologist for chronic esophagitis and chronic duodenitis. ELISA revealed contamination with *Toxocara* and *Giardia lamblia*; therapy with albendazole was administrated on an outpatient basis. However, the carriage of Toxocara continued. A repeated course of treatment was conducted in adolescence, but the antibody titer remained. Further courses of therapy were canceled, and *Toxocara* IgG antibody carriage was diagnosed. When the patient was 15, follow-up examination at the gastroenterology department revealed hydronephrosis of the nonfunctioning right kidney. Previously, there were no complaints or clinical manifestations indicating the damage to the urinary organs; urinalysis was unremarkable; blood pressure was normal.

In the course of further examination, urography showed a nonfunctioning right kidney; the excretory function of the left kidney was maintained. Cystography did not reveal any reflux. The patient underwent right nephrectomy.

Findings of the histology exam revealed a kidney with enlarged pelvis cups and the presence of cavities filled with fluid in the medulla and partly in the cortical layer. The capsule of the kidney was thickened by sclerosis. Renal glomeruli demonstrated fibrosis of the capsule with thickening, focal sclerosis of individual glomeruli, and singular glomerular cysts. Multiple, large-sized granulomas with necrosis in the center, surrounded by epithelioid cells and lymphocytes, including Pirogov-Langhans giant cells and eosinophils, were found mainly in the cortical layer (**Figures 1–4**).

Smaller granulomas showed fibrosis without central necrosis. Hyaline-droplet dystrophy was noted in the convoluted tubules. Sclerosis was detected in the vessels, diffuse lymphocellular infiltration and foci of fibrosis were observed in the stroma.

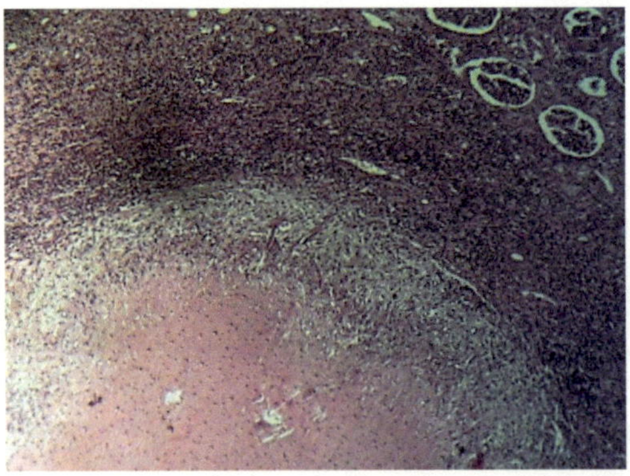

Figure 1.
Medium-sized granuloma and peripheral lymphocytic infiltration. Renal glomeruli with edema of the mesangium are seen in the upper part.

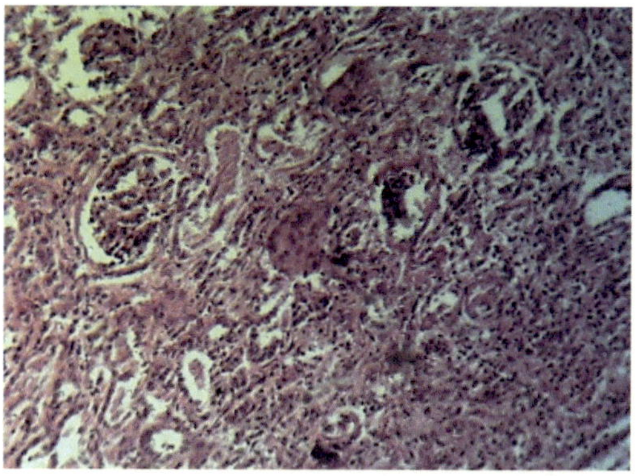

Figure 2.
A giant multinucleated cell in the center. To the left and to the right, there are renal glomeruli with edema, tubules with dystrophic changes, and the stroma replete with lymphoid infiltration.

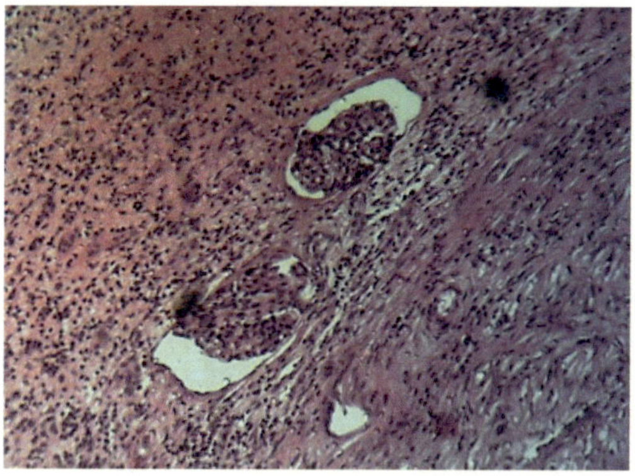

Figure 3.
The giant granuloma; two glomeruli with marked mesangial edema are on top. Renal tissue with pronounced lymphoid infiltration.

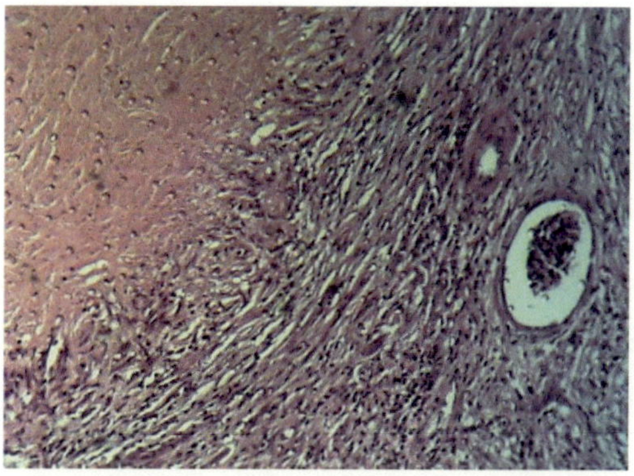

Figure 4.
Granuloma with surrounding infiltration. A granuloma with a necrotic focus in the center. On the periphery, there is a proliferation of connective tissue fibers with mildly expressed lymphocytic infiltration (a marker of chronic inflammation).

2. Granulomatous nephritis resulted in nephrosclerosis

Granulomas had large central foci of necrosis with features of organization. There was no presence of microorganisms; the absence of microorganisms could be related to the remoteness of the process.

The detection of granulomatous nephritis during histological examination prompted an extended diagnostic screening in order to seek the etiology of the disease.

On examination, the patient's condition was satisfactory. The patient complained of pain in the right leg with loss of sensitivity. The girl was asthenic; her height was 185 cm, weight 57 kg, and BMI 16.65. The subcutaneous fat layer was poorly developed. Her skin was dry overall with fading rashes of atopic dermatitis on the chest and extremities.

The findings of the ultrasound examination documented that the right kidney had been removed. The left kidney had compensatory enlargement. Cortical-medullary differentiation was preserved; there was a moderate amount of hyperechoic signals and a thin hyperechoic rim around the pyramids. Functional bend of the gallbladder was found. Structure of the pancreas was moderately inhomogeneous.

MRI of the lumbosacral part of the spinal column and cauda equina revealed scoliosis and degenerative-dystrophic changes in the intervertebral discs of the lumbosacral spine, sacralization of L5, spina bifida S1–S3, and no MRI signs of organic pathology of cauda equina.

During the observation period, CBC revealed moderate leukocytosis (up to 11.5×10^9/l), mild anemia (maximum hemoglobin reduction to 103 g/l), and an intermittent increase in ESR to 27–28 mm/hour.

Biochemical blood analysis showed no pathological changes, except for an increased level of CRP up to 7.44 mg/l. Protein, fat, mineral metabolism, as well as the level of enzymes were normal.

For this patient we ruled out autoimmune diseases (rheumatoid factor 1.4 IU/l, ASLO 141.5 IU/l, antibodies to DNA, and antibodies to extractable nuclear antigens were not detected), TORCH infections, viral hepatitis C, HIV infection, and tuberculosis.

We also excluded parasitic diseases such as echinococcosis, opisthorchiasis, trichinosis, and brucellosis.

Helminthic eggs were not found. Blood test for *Toxocara* antibodies was slightly positive 1:200.

Clinical urinalysis revealed traces of protein (daily protein excretion—negative), up to 10 leukocytes per hpf and up to 3–5 erythrocytes per hpf (in isolated tests).

Oxaluria was detected (excretion of 98.4 mg/day, daily diuresis of 2000 ml). Urate excretion was normal (2.14 mmol/day).

The glomerular filtration rate by the Schwartz formula was 102 ml/min.

Final diagnosis was single left kidney and loss of renal concentration ability. The condition after surgical treatment (right nephrectomy in January 2016, hydronephrosis stage 5 with absence of right kidney function, morphologically: granulomatous interstitial nephritis resulting in nephrosclerosis).

She had atopic dermatitis; chronic gastroduodenitis; erosive gastritis Hp (+/−); gastroesophageal reflux disease; biliary dysfunction reactive pancreatic changes; oxaluria; juvenile osteochondrosis; sacralization of L5; spina bifida S1–S3; neuritis of the sciatic nerve; juvenile kyphosis; thoracolumbar scoliosis, grade 2; body weight deficit, grade 1; mild myopia; chronic subcompensated tonsillitis; and carriage of *Toxocara* antibodies.

This clinical case was peculiar due to the comorbidity of the patient and the impossibility of accurate identification of the main etiologic agent of GIN.

Our patient was diagnosed with toxocariasis at the age of 3 years, when she received anthelmintic treatment; however, the results of immunological studies showed that *Toxocara* carriage continued. *Toxocara canis* is a large roundworm, the source of which is dogs or less commonly cats. Toxocariasis is characterized by a long-term recurrent course with damage to organs and systems based on immunopathic processes [11]. The clinical picture may include general symptoms of infectious toxic syndrome, subfebrile condition, cough, and enlargement of the liver and lymph nodes. Systemic forms of toxocariasis may damage the heart, the pancreas, and the central nervous system (resulting in epileptic seizures). From a pathomorphological point of view, toxocariasis causes disseminated eosinophilic granulomatosis [11]. There is no conclusive data connecting parasitosis with renal damage; but there are reported cases of experimental models [11] and individual case reports, mainly in the form of nephrotic syndrome [11–13].

For 1 and 1/2 years, the patient suffered from atopic dermatitis and periodic exacerbations. Nephrologists from St. Petersburg described the formation of granulomas from epithelioid histiocytes and giant cells in allergic types of acute interstitial nephritis; in addition to the aforementioned, tuberculosis, sarcoidosis, Wegener's granulomatosis, and berylliosis were excluded in our patient [14]. An association between atopic diseases and idiopathic nephrotic syndrome and minimal change glomerulonephritis has also been described [15, 16]. Perhaps, the peculiarities of the individual response of the immune system contribute to an increased risk of atopy and immunopathic diseases of the kidneys. However, in the patient's medical notes, there are no records of acute interstitial nephritis and any episode of renal failure in the past, and nephromegaly was discovered accidentally.

The pathology of the gastrointestinal tract, except for Crohn's disease, can hardly be the cause of GIN.

Therefore, though it is difficult to identify the importance of comorbidity as the cause of GIN, we assumed that infection from *Toxocara* carriage is etiologically responsible for the development of GIN in our patient.

Granulomatous interstitial nephritis can be a manifestation of systemic diseases, such as Wegener's granulomatosis, Crohn's disease [17], and sarcoidosis. Usually, renal damage in sarcoidosis is associated with nephrocalcinosis, hypercalciuria, or urolithiasis [4]. The development of granulomatous inflammation of the kidneys is considered to be rare, with a frequency of 0.7–30% [18]. However, the proportion of sarcoidosis in the etiological structure of GIN can be from 9 to 29% [6]. In the study conducted by Oliveira et al., sarcoidosis with extrarenal damage was detected in 38% of patients, and 24% of patients had sarcoidosis with only renal damage [19]. In the literature, we found cases wherein the GIN preceded the diagnosis of sarcoidosis [1, 4]. Stehlé et al. reported that in 23% of cases, glomerulopathy supported the diagnosis of sarcoidosis, with an average delay of 8 years in diagnosing it [20]. According to Bagnasco, the results of a biopsy of a native kidney in 51 patients with sarcoidosis showed that GIN was the most common finding (19 cases, 37%) [18]. Similar data on the prevalence of GIN in sarcoidosis (approximately 30%) were obtained in a study conducted by Löffler et al. [21].

Due to the rarity of the disease, the degree of influence of GIN in sarcoidosis on the disease progression up to the terminal stage of CKD remains in question. There are no clinical recommendations for the therapy of renal sarcoidosis, though the use of glucocorticoids is considered the standard treatment.

We had another clinical case which was a type of granulomatous kidney disease associated with a rare form of primary immunodeficiency—chronic granulomatous disease (OMIM 233,670, 233,690, 233,700, 233,710, 306,400, 613,960). This disease is characterized by increased vulnerability to severe bacterial and fungal infections (most often *Staphylococcus aureus* and *Aspergillus* spp) and granuloma formation.

The cause of the disease is a mutation of one of five genes encoding phagocyte nicotinamide adenine dinucleotide phosphate (NADPH) oxidase subunits. The mutation of the CYBB gene (Xp21.1) is detected in most cases. The mechanism of granuloma formation is not clear, but in this disease abnormally long activation of neutrophils in inflammation foci is noted, which leads to chronic inflammation [22]. Most often, granulomatous damage involves the skin, lymph nodes, gastrointestinal tract, and liver [23]. Usually, the disease is diagnosed within the first 5 years of life; however, some cases presenting in adulthood have also been reported [23, 24].

This disease presented in a boy, who manifested all the typical symptoms. This 16-year-old boy was sick from birth. He was diagnosed with primary immunodeficiency and chronic granulomatous disease (missense mutation in exon 1 J of the CYBB gene in the hemizygous state: c.1169 > T,CCC > CTC, p.Pro390Leu).

He had a positive family history. The patient's mother suffered from pyelonephritis and arthritis. Her three brothers died in childhood: one of them died of systemic lupus erythematosus at the age of 9, the second from respiratory infection when he was 1.5 years old, and the third at 3 months (the cause unknown). Chronic granulomatous disease had not been diagnosed due to the lack of diagnostic methods at that time; however, the association of the disease with autoimmune disorders and severe life-threatening infections at an early age was characteristic of the disease [25–27].

At the age of 1 year, our patient had contact with a TBC patient; he was operated for tuberculoma when he was 6 years old.

Starting with the second year of life, the child suffered from recurrent bacterial infections in variable locations, which were typical of chronic granulomatous disease, paronychia, balanoposthitis, purulent otitis media, pneumonia, purulent lymphadenitis, furunculosis, abscesses of the anterior abdominal wall, and liver abscesses with inoculation of mainly catalase-positive microorganisms (characteristic of granulomatous disease) [28, 29]. The patient had no infections of fungal etiology.

When the patient was 5 years of age, a secondary immunodeficiency condition was suspected, but no further examinations were carried out. The diagnosis of primary immunodeficiency was made at the age of 14 years; the genetic test was carried out at the age of 17 years.

In addition to infectious complications, the patient also had inflammatory complications affecting the gastrointestinal tract in the form of chronic gastroduodenitis, although intestinal lesions are considered more frequent [30–32].

Renal damage in chronic granulomatous disease is frequent and is usually associated with obstruction and urinary tract infections [30, 31]. However, there are reported cases of glomerulonephritis associated with granulomatous disease [33].

Our patient had various types of urinary tract problems, namely, episodes of urinary tract infection since the age of 5 years; diagnosis of acute glomerulonephritis with nephritic syndrome when he was 11 years old; urolithiasis since the age of 14 years and secondary chronic glomerulonephritis, hematuric form with preserved renal function; nephrobiopsy revealing IgA nephropathy; segmental and complete glomerulosclerosis; expressed tubular fibrosis; arteriosclerosis; and diffuse chronic tubulointerstitial nephritis. The patient has had stage 2 chronic kidney disease (GFR 44–61 ml/min) to date, with moderate positive dynamic and response to therapy with mycophenolate mofetil.

3. Conclusion

In conclusion, although GIN is rare, it is a disease most probably underestimated in frequency in pediatric practice; the variety of etiological causes of GIN, the absence of noninvasive diagnostic methods, as well as the possibility of development of GIN in multiple pathologies and genetic syndromes render the task of diagnosis difficult for the physician. Moreover, the lack of clinical guidelines for diagnosis and management is another issue which generally complicates treatment and leads to a poor renal prognosis.

Author details

Galina Makovetskaya, Lilia Mazur and Elena Balashova*
Samara State Medical University, Samara, Russia

*Address all correspondence to: mine22@yandex.ru

References

[1] Nikitina EN, Povilaytite PE, Matsionis AE. Case of extrapulmonary sarcoidosis with renal injury. Nephrology. 2014;5(18):76-79

[2] Aleckovic-Halilovic M, Nel D, Woywodt A. Granulomatous interstitial nephritis: A chameleon in a globalized world. Clinical Kidney Journal. 2015;**8**(5):511-515. DOI: 10.1093/ckj/sfv092

[3] Jung JH, Kang KP, Kim W, Kwang S, Lee S. Nonsteroidal antiinflammatory drug induced acute granulomatous interstitial nephritis. BMC Research Notes. 2015;**8**:793. DOI: 10.1186/s13104-015-1788-2

[4] Shah S, Carter-Monroe N, Atta MG. Granulomatous interstitial nephritis. Clinical Kidney Journal. 2015;**8**(5):516-523. DOI: 10.1093/ckj/sfv053

[5] Churilina AV, Masyuta DI, Manzheleev GN, Artemenko SP. Interstitial nephritis in children. Etiological aspects (review of foreign literature). International Journal of Medicine. 2013;**6**(1):62-66

[6] Ogura M, Kagami S, Nakao M, Kono M, Kanetsuna Y, Hosoya T. Fungal granulomatous interstitial nephritis presenting as acute kidney injury diagnosed by renal histology including PCR assay. Clinical Kidney Journal. 2012;**5**(5):459-462. DOI: 10.1093/ckj/sfs103

[7] Naidu GD, Ram R, Swarnalatha G, Uppin M, Prayaga AK, Dakshinamurty KV. Granulomatous interstitial nephritis: Our experience of 14 patients. Indian Journal of Nephrology. 2013;**23**(6):415-418. DOI: 10.4103/0971-4065.120336

[8] Nel D. A retrospective review of Granulomatous Interstitial Nephritis (GIN) amongst HIV-infected patients at Groote Schuur Hospital Cape Town [Doctoral thesis]. Cape Town: Faculty of Health Sciences, University of Cape Town; 2014

[9] Milosevski-Lomic G, Markovic-Lipkovski J, Paripovic KMD, Spasojevic-Dimitrijeva B, Peco-Antic A. Granulomatous interstitial nephritis associated with influenza A: H1N1 infection: A case report. Srpski Arhiv za Celokupno Lekarstvo. 2016;**144**(3-4):215-218

[10] Balafa O, Liapis G, Duni A, Xiromeriti S, Kalaitzidis R, Elisaf M. An unusual case of acute kidney injury–idiopathic granulomatous tubulointerstitial nephritis. Clinical Nephrology. 2015;**84**(4):247-250. DOI: 10.5414/CN108543

[11] Nikulin TY, Pchelnikov YV, Baklanova MS, Pchelnikova EF. Renal Pathology in Children Caused by Toxocariasis. Protection of Maternal and Child Health. 2008;**2**(12):60-64

[12] Zotos PG, Psimenou E, Roussou M, Kontogiannis S, Panoutsopoulos A, Dimopoulos A-M. Nephrotic syndrome as a manifestation of Toxocara canis infection. Nephrology, Dialysis, Transplantation. 2006;**21**:2676. DOI: 10.1093/ndt/gfl224

[13] Shetty AK, Aviles DH. Nephrotic syndrome associated with/Toxocara canis/infection. Annals of Tropical Paediatrics. 1999;**19**(3):297-300

[14] Materials for the satellite lecture ourse "Vascular and interstitial kidney disease." In: XIII St. Petersburg Nephrology Seminar; St. Petersburg; 12-13 June 2005. 20 p

[15] Abdel-Hafez M, Shimada M, Lee PY, Johnson RJ, Garin EH. Idiopathic nephrotic syndrome and atopy: Is there a common link? American Journal of

Kidney Diseases. 2009;**54**(5):945-953. DOI: 10.1053/j.ajkd.2009.03.019

[16] Wei C-C, Lin C-L, Shen T-C, Sung F-C. Occurrence of common allergic diseases in children with idiopathic nephrotic syndrome. Journal of Epidemiology. 2015;**25**(5):370-377. DOI: 10.2188/jea.JE20140167

[17] Timmermans SAMEG, Christiaans MHL, Abdul-Hamid MA, Stifft F, Damoiseaux JGMC, van Paassen P. Granulomatous interstitial nephritis and Crohn's disease. Clinical Kidney Journal. 2016;**9**(4):556-559. DOI: 10.1093/ckj/sfw041

[18] Bagnasco SM, Gottipati S, Kraus E, Alachkar N, Montgomery RA, Racusen LC, et al. Sarcoidosis in native and transplanted kidneys: Incidence, pathologic findings, and clinical course. In: Camussi G, editor. PLoS One. 2014;**9**(10):e110778. DOI: 10.1371/journal.pone.0110778

[19] Oliveira B, Jayawardene S, Shah S. Single-centre experience of granulomatous interstitial nephritis—time for a new approach? Clinical Kidney Journal. 2017;**10**(2):249-254. DOI: 10.1093/ckj/sfw119

[20] Stehlé T, Joly D, Vanhille P, Boffa J-J, Remy P, Mesnard L, et al. Clinicopathological study of glomerular diseases associated with sarcoidosis: A multicenter study. Orphanet Journal of Rare Diseases. 2013;**8**:65. DOI: 10.1186/1750-1172-8-65

[21] Löffler U, Tuleweit A, Waldherr R, Uppenkamp M, Bergner R. Renal sarcoidosis: Epidemiological and follow-up data in a cohort of 27 patients. Sarcoidosis, Vasculitis, and Diffuse Lung Diseases. 2015;**4**(31):306-315

[22] Katsuya Y, Hojo M, Kawai S, Kawai T, Onodera M, Sugiyama H. Chronic granulomatous disease with pulmonary mass-like opacities secondary to hypersensitivity pneumonitis: A case report. Journal of Medical Case Reports. 2014;**8**:242. DOI: 10.1186/1752-1947-8-242

[23] Schwenkenbecher P, Neyazi A, Donnerstag F, Donnerstag F, Ringshausen FC, Jacobs R, et al. Chronic granulomatous disease first diagnosed in adulthood presenting with spinal cord infection. Frontiers in Immunology. 2018;**9**:1258. DOI: 10.3389/fimmu.2018.01258

[24] Yamashita Y, Kimura T, Tanaka N, Yazaki M, Itagaki T, Joshita S, et al. Salmonella enteritidis cholecystitis with chronic granulomatous disease. IDCases. 2018;**12**:49-52. DOI: 10.1016/j.idcr.2018.03.012

[25] Cale CM, Morton L, Goldblatt D. Cutaneous and other lupus-like symptoms in carriers of X-linked chronic granulomatous disease: Incidence and autoimmune serology. Clinical and Experimental Immunology. 2007;**148**(1):79-84. DOI: 10.1111/j.1365-2249.2007.03321.x

[26] Stalder J, Dreno B, Bureau B, Hakim J. Discoid lupus erythematosus-like lesions in an autosomal form of chronic granulomatous disease. British Journal of Dermatology. 1986;**114**:251-254. DOI: 10.1111/j.1365-2133.1986.tb02805.x

[27] Lee BW, Yap HK. Polyarthritis resembling juvenile rheumatoid arthritis in a girl with chronic granulomatous disease. Arthritis and Rheumatism. 1994;**37**:773-776. DOI: 10.1002/art.1780370524

[28] Soler-Palacín P, Margareto C, Llobet P, Asensio O, Hernández M, Caragol I, et al. Chronic granulomatous disease in pediatric patients: 25 years of experience. Allergol Immunopathol (Madr). 2007;**35**:83-89. DOI: 10.1157/13106774

[29] Yu JE, Azar AE, Chong HJ, Jongco AM, Prince BT. Considerations in the

diagnosis of chronic granulomatous disease. Journal of the Pediatric Infectious Diseases Society. 2018;7(Suppl 1):S6-S11. DOI: 10.1093/jpids/piy007

[30] Arnold DE, Heimall JR. A review of chronic granulomatous disease. Advances in Therapy. 2017;**34**(12):2543-2557. DOI: 10.1007/s12325-017-0636-2

[31] Henrickson SE, Jongco AM, Thomsen KF, Garabedian EK, Thomsen IP. Noninfectious manifestations and complications of chronic granulomatous disease. Journal of the Pediatric Infectious Diseases Society. 2018;7(Suppl 1):S18-S24. DOI: 10.1093/jpids/piy014

[32] Barbato M, Ragusa G, Civitelli F, Marcheggiano A, Di Nardo G, Iacobini M, et al. Chronic granulomatous disease mimicking early-onset Crohn's disease with cutaneous manifestations. BMC Pediatrics. 2014;**14**:156. DOI: 10.1186/1471-2431-14-156

[33] Frifelt JJ, Schønheyder H, Valerius NH, Strate M, Starklint H. Chronic granulomatous disease associated with chronic glomerulonephritis. Acta Paediatrica Scandinavica. 1985;**74**(1):152-157

Chapter 7

Cardiac Sarcoidosis

Jhan Carlos Altamar Castillo and Miguel Jose Tejeda Camargo

Abstract

Sarcoidosis is a systemic disease of unknown origin characterized by the infiltration of non-necrotizing granulomas that can affect any organ. The presentation of cardiac involvement can range from slight infiltration to complete atrioventricular block, ventricular arrhythmia, or cardiac failure. The diagnosis requires a high index of suspicion; approach to treatment depends upon the presence, or absence, of extracardiac sarcoidosis; sometimes a biopsy of the myocardial tissue is the only way to obtain an accurate diagnosis. Nuclear magnetic resonance imaging is the imaging technique which can provide information useful in diagnosis of this condition. If there is active inflammation, the fundamental form of treatment is immunosuppression therapy. Other concomitant treatments can be required such as the implantation of devices or modulation of arrhythmias. The prognosis is conditioned depending upon the extent of the disease and response to the therapy.

Keywords: sarcoidosis, nuclear magnetic resonance imaging, cardiac block, cardiac failure, arrhythmias, immunosuppression

1. Introduction

Sarcoidosis is a systemic disease of unknown origin characterized by infiltration of non-necrotizing granulomas. This disease can affect any organ, including the heart. The heart can be involved to a variable extent depending on the area studied [1]. The ACCES study reported about 95% of findings compatible with cardiac involvement [2]. Others report mainly pulmonary involvement. Studies in Japan report cardiac infiltration up to 25% in contrast with the European studies in which the prevalence ranges from 2 to 7% [3].

2. Epidemiology

Sarcoidosis has a worldwide prevalence of 4.7–64 per 100,000 individuals; the highest rates are found in Northern Europe and among Afro-Americans, predominantly in females [4]. The real prevalence of cardiac sarcoidosis is unknown. In some cases, it can be isolated without extracardiac involvement and in others can have no symptoms; the average age for this disease is 50 [5]. When the clinical behaviors of isolated cardiac sarcoidosis among the group of patients who also register extracardiac compromise are compared, it is found that patients who have the disease confined to the heart exhibit a higher prevalence of complete block of the right branch, delayed myocardial enhancement, and less elevation of the angiotensin-converting enzyme in serum, as they are clinically very similar in their presentation.

3. Pathogenesis

This is a multisystem condition, of unknown etiology, which affects the lungs in most patients (90%) and usually involves the nodes and mediastinum. Cardiac involvement varies according to the population studied and can reach up to 25% [3]. The typical histological feature is the presence of non-necrotizing granuloma (see **Figure 1**) [6] with a central area rich in macrophages, epithelial cells, giant multinucleated cells, and T CD4-positive lymphocytes. In the periphery, there is an abundant population of T CD8 and CD4 lymphocytes, mast cells, and fibroblasts [7]. The origin of this condition is unknown, but one of the theories proposed is antigenic stimulation due to occupational and environmental exposure and infectious agents such as mycobacteria [8].

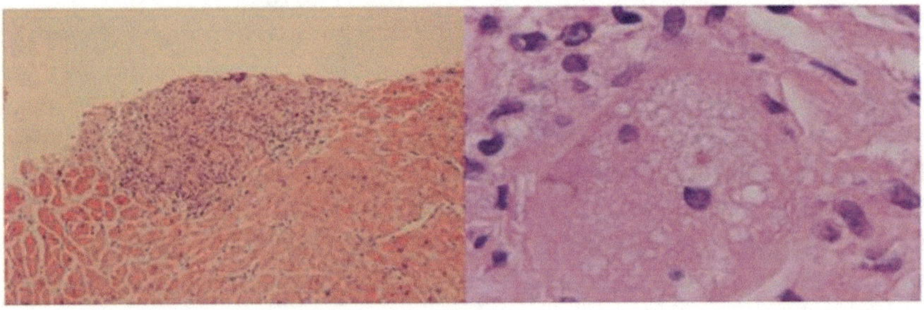

Figure 1.
Cardiac tissue biopsy. Fragments of myocardium can be observed with compromise due to multiple epithelial, non-necrotizing, focal, and coalesced granules, which involve about 30% of the tissue analyzed. The granules contain numerous multinucleated giant cells and, in the confluent areas, are associated with interstitial fibrosis. Stains were negative for mycobacteria and fungi.

4. Clinical manifestations

The manifestations of sarcoidosis vary and depend on the presence or absence of extracardiac compromise, extension, localization, and activity. The majority of heart signs and symptoms are subsequent to arrhythmia, anomalies in atrioventricular conduction, and ventricular arrhythmia (including sudden death) as well as cardiac failure [4]. A less frequent clinical presentation is vasculitis of the coronary arteries. The clinical presentation ranges from palpitations, dyspnea, chest pain, to cardiorespiratory arrest.

Anomalies in atrioventricular conduction are the most frequent manifestation of cardiovascular compromise. They can have a variable clinical presentation that ranges from fixed prolongation of the PR interval (atrioventricular block degree 1) to the presence of branch blocks and in more advanced cases complete atrioventricular block. A prospective study identified that up to 34% of patients with atrioventricular block who were younger than 60 years old, without an apparently clear cause, were eventually diagnosed with sarcoidosis [9], the reason this entity should always be suspected in young patients who present with these alterations without an evident etiology.

The second form of presentation is ventricular arrhythmias which include the presence of premature ventricular complexes and ventricular tachycardia (sustained and non-sustained), mostly subsequent to an increase in cardiac automatism or a reentrant mechanism around the scar caused by granulomas in the myocardium. This type of compromise takes place in ~30% of patients [5]; even these arrhythmias can be the first manifestation of sarcoidosis [6].

Another form of presentation of arrhythmia is supraventricular tachycardia. In a retrospective study of 100 cases, the global prevalence of these arrhythmias was 32%, with auricular fibrillation being the most frequently detected arrhythmia; the methods used for detection were continuous electrocardiogram, Holter monitoring devices, and electrophysiological studies. The majority of patients were asymptomatic (96%), and after atrial fibrillation, in order of frequency, they had atrial tachycardia and atrial flutter. The presence of diastolic dysfunction, increase in the size of the left atrium, and arterial hypertension were the most important factors in the multivariate analysis [10].

Sudden death is a more unusual situation in cardiac sarcoidosis, but when it takes place, it is usually subsequent to severe malfunction in atrioventricular conduction or ventricular arrhythmia. It seems that the presence of delayed enhancement with gadolinium in nuclear magnetic resonance imaging correlated with this outcome; however, these findings are yet to be confirmed.

In some people, cardiac failure can be the main manifestation, followed by dyspnea, orthopnea, and lower limb edema [11]. The right or left ventricular function may be compromised; there may be disorders of segmental or global contractility, as well as valvular compromise, and pulmonary hypertension [12]. There should be a high degree of suspicion regarding this condition, principally when there is a manifest extrapulmonary clinical picture or antecedents of such condition are not present.

The involvement of the epicardial coronary arteries is rare; however, there are reports of cases of vasculitis presenting as acute coronary syndrome and even spontaneous dissection of the coronary arteries, cardiac tamponade, and death in patients without any known antecedents of cardiac sarcoidosis [13, 14].

5. Diagnosis

The diagnosis of this condition in particular starts with a high index of suspicion; other possible causes must not be overlooked, taking into consideration the wide clinical spectrum of this pathology. The treatment of this condition requires a significant medical effort with clinical imaging and, in many cases, histological correlation.

Cardiac compromise due to sarcoidosis should be suspected when the following conditions take place in which the most frequent causes are excluded [15]:

- Advanced atrioventricular block in patients younger than 60 years old
- Cardiac failure
- Ventricular arrhythmia

In addition, clinical suspicion should be higher in all patients with antecedents of extracardiac sarcoidosis that occurred with a cardiovascular symptom such as syncope, arrhythmias, or cardiac insufficiency.

Thus, the diagnosis of this pathology starts with clinical suspicion generated after a detailed medical record and an exhaustive physical exam of those conditions that might explain the current clinical picture is ruled out and identification of extracardiac compromise is found to be due to sarcoidosis.

The use of complementary studies should follow a logical sequence that supports or rules out the suspicion generated in the clinic. The following complementary tests must be performed:

5.1 Chest image

Chest image continues to be the initial study; it is used to identify the typical anomalies of cardiac sarcoidosis; chest images are reported as abnormal in up to 95% of the cases [16] reserving high-resolution tomography for those cases in which the thorax image is normal or presents atypical findings. Image analysis should always take into consideration the multiple differential diagnoses, infections, or conditions that might compromise the lung in a similar way [17].

5.2 Electrocardiogram and Holter

The electrocardiogram is abnormal in the majority of patients with symptomatic cardiac sarcoidosis, compared with patients that have a silent compromise in which the abnormality does not go above 9% [4, 18].

In the screening of asymptomatic patients with extracardiac sarcoidosis confirmed via biopsy [19], the most suggestive findings are:

- Right or left branch block
- One or more signals of a signal-averaged ECG
- One or more premature ventricular complexes
- Presence of Q wave in two or more adjacent leads in the absence of myocardial infarction
- Fragmented QRS in two or more adjacent leads in the absence of myocardial infarction
- Atrial arrhythmia (atrial tachycardia or atrial fibrillation)

Table 1 summarizes the ECG manifestations with variable prevalence according to the course of the cardiac sarcoidosis [19].

As noted before, up to 34% of cases show malfunction in atrioventricular conduction (57% of patients being reversible in some series after immunosuppression therapy) [19]. Other alterations identified are changes in the ST T wave and rarely epsilon waves [4].

Ambulatory electrocardiographic monitoring which continues for 24–48 h (Holter) is useful for identification of arrhythmias, as well as their response to treatment [20].

5.3 Echocardiogram

The echocardiographic findings are diverse with low sensitivity and specificity; however, they are useful for follow-up of patients to monitor progression of the disease [3]. The alterations that stand out include anomalies of the segmental and global contractility (usually following a non-coronary epicardial pattern), thickening or thinning of the interventricular septum (especially toward the base), diastolic dysfunction, and ventricular hypertrophy which can simulate a hypertrophic cardiomyopathy and aneurysms [4]. In recent studies, interest has grown in utility of longitudinal deformity of the left ventricle via Speckle-tracking analysis to identify patients with cardiac sarcoidosis; this can be a useful tool in the early diagnosis and the follow-up of the disease [21].

Presentation	Prevalence (%)
Atrioventricular block	26–67
Bundle block	12–61
Atrial arrhythmias	23–25
Ventricular arrhythmias	11–73

Table 1.
Prevalence of ECG abnormalities.

5.4 Advanced cardiovascular imaging

5.4.1 Nuclear magnetic resonance imaging

Nuclear magnetic resonance imaging is one of the most useful imaging techniques for the assessment of cardiac sarcoidosis. There is no pattern that can be defined as typical; however, the delayed enhancement of the gadolinium is patched (and does not follow a vascular pattern); it compromises the myocardium and the subepicardium, unlike acute myocardial infraction that compromises the subendocardium; it usually affects the basal segments of the septum and the inferolateral wall. Left ventricle involvement is more common. Transmural and right ventricle compromise is infrequent; however, these findings do not rule out the presence of the cardiac sarcoidosis. Some series report a negative predictive value up to 100% with epidemiological limitations with respect to the gold pattern. For this reason, although a negative cardiac resonance image is not common, cardiac compromise due to this pathology cannot be disregarded, especially if the probability and clinical suspicion are high [22, 23]. The superiority of the cardiac nuclear magnetic resonance imaging in the diagnosis of sarcoidosis was proven by Ichinose et al. [24]; he found sensitivity from 75 to 100% and specificity from 39 to 78%. He showed that the NMRI is superior to SPECT with thallium and gallium [25]. The increase in the T2 signal correlated in some subjects with inflammation and major adverse events; NMRI continues to be studied [20, 22]. The limitations of NMRI include patients with implanted cardiac devices (relative), chronic renal disease (stage 4/5), and claustrophobia.

5.4.2 Fluorodeoxyglucose positron 18 emission tomography

This imaging technique is useful in cardiac sarcoidosis for the identification of possible areas with active inflammatory processes; an algorithm has been proposed as a response test to treatment [3]. As a diagnostic guide, a meta-analysis concluded 89% sensibility and 78% specificity; however, these results should be viewed with caution and with the diagnostic criteria used as a pattern [26].

Advanced cardiovascular imaging is advised in the following clinical contexts [27]: Patients with extracardiac compromise

- Presence of more than one of the following symptoms: 2 weeks + of palpitations, pre-syncope, or syncope

- One or more of the following anomalies in the electrocardiogram: complete block of right or left branch, presence of unexplained pathologic Q waves in two or more leads, atrioventricular block at any degree of severity, and sustained or non-sustained ventricular tachycardia

- One or more of the following echocardiographic anomalies: anomalies in the regional movement of a wall, ventricular aneurysm, thinning of the interventricular septum (basal segment), and ejection fraction of the left ventricle below 50%

Patients without extracardiac compromise

- Atrioventricular block second-degree Mobitz II or third degree in adults younger than 60 years old without an evident cause
- Monomorphic ventricular tachycardia without a clear cause

5.5 Biomarkers

The angiotensin-converting enzyme has been found to be high in 75% of the patients with non-treated sarcoidosis, it does not have much diagnostic value due to its low sensitivity and specificity, and multiple conditions such as diabetes mellitus, tuberculosis, hyperthyroidism, and lung cancer, among other entities, can alter its levels [28]. The measurement of the soluble receptor of interleukin 2 has been proposed as an inflammatory marker in patients with extrapulmonary disease [28]; more studies are needed to assess its use in the clinical setting.

5.6 Endomyocardial biopsy

Being an invasive procedure and considering that sarcoidosis is usually a disease with multisystem compromise, it is preferred to identify a possible extracardiac site for biopsy and histological studies (lymph nodes or lungs). In cases in which the histological tests are not conclusive or there is only cardiac compromise, the endomyocardial biopsy becomes important in the diagnosis of this condition. The diagnostic performance of a blind biopsy is 25% [29] increasing to 50% when guided by images or electroanatomic mapping; this is logical when taking into consideration the multifocal nature of the infiltration [30, 31].

6. Diagnostic criteria

There is no global consensus accepted for the diagnosis of cardiac sarcoidosis. In 2014 The European Heart Rate Society (HRS) published a consensus for the histological and clinical diagnosis of sarcoidosis with cardiac compromise which is shown in **Table 2** [27].

7. Differential diagnostic

The differential diagnosis of this condition is difficult considering all the pathologies that can manifest in a similar form. The complete medical record and the physical exam are the most important ways to make a diagnostic approach.

8. Management

The medical and interventional management in sarcoidosis requires interaction of a multidisciplinary team that includes a cardiologist, electrophysiologist, rheumatologist, pneumologist, and other specialists.

Histological diagnosis of myocardial tissue
Presence of granuloma not classified in the histological exam of the myocardial tissue without an alternative identified cause (including staining for microorganisms)
Clinical diagnosis (invasive studies and noninvasive): recognized as probable
a. Histological diagnosis of extracardiac sarcoidosis
b. One or more of the following:
I. Cardiac block or cardiomyopathy with response to immunosuppression therapy with steroids
II. Ejection fraction of the left ventricle reduced in an unexplainable form (<40%)
III. Sustained ventricular tachycardia with no clear cause (spontaneous or induced)
IV. Atrioventricular block second-degree Mobitz II or cardiac block third degree
V. Irregular captation in a positron emission heart tomography (a consistent pattern with cardiac sarcoidosis)
VI. Delayed enhancement with gadolinium in a cardiac nuclear magnetic resonance (in a pattern consistent with cardiac sarcoidosis)
VII. Positive gallium captation (in a pattern consistent with cardiac sarcoidosis)
c. Other causes of the cardiac manifestations have been reasonably excluded

Table 2.
Diagnostic criteria for sarcoidosis (HRS) 2014.

Left ventricular dysfunction and evidence of myocardial inflammation
Cardiac block Mobitz II and degree III and evidence of myocardial inflammation
Sustained ventricular arrhythmia and evidence of myocardial inflammation
Non-sustained ventricular arrhythmia and frequent ventricular ectopy and evidence of myocardial inflammation

Table 3.
Indication of immunosuppression therapy.

All patients with cardiac sarcoidosis should have a proper control of cardiovascular risk factors, management of cardiac failure in case it occurs, treatment of ventricular arrhythmias and atrioventricular conduction malfunction, as well as immunosuppression therapy.

Immunosuppression therapy is prescribed in all patients with cardiac sarcoidosis. The criteria shown in **Table 3** should be fulfilled [27]. Corticosteroids (prednisolone goes from 30 to 40 mg/day) [32] and the clinical response should be assessed 1–3 months after the starting treatment. The dosage should be reduced gradually, as low as 5–15 mg/day, until completing 9–12 months of sustained treatment. The patients should undergo clinical follow-up for up to 3 years after the therapy to identify relapse. Other therapies (second or third line) include methotrexate, infliximab, cyclophosphamide, and azathioprine, used in refractory cases or when steroids adverse effects are not tolerated. In immunosuppression treatment it is essential to identify the inflamed myocardium via histological study or imaging. It is here where fluorodeoxyglucose positron 18 emission tomography becomes important. It is worth noting this is proposed as a follow-up strategy to define which patients should continue with or discontinue therapy [26, 27].

Table 4 lists the recommendations by consensus for the management of arrhythmias related to cardiac sarcoidosis [4, 27].

Management of conduction malfunctions	
The implantation of a device can be useful in patients with cardiac sarcoidosis with stimulation indication, even if the atrioventricular block is reverted transiently	IIa
Immunosuppression can be useful in patients with cardiac sarcoidosis with atrioventricular block second degree (Mobitz II) or third degree	IIa
The implantation of a cardioverter can be useful in patients with cardiac sarcoidosis and an indication of permanent implantation of a pacemaker	IIa
Management of ventricular arrhythmias	
The assessment of myocardial inflammation via fluorodeoxyglucose positron 18 emission tomography can be useful in patients with cardiac sarcoidosis with ventricular arrhythmias	IIa
Immunosuppression can be useful in patients with cardiac sarcoidosis with ventricular arrhythmias and evidence of myocardial inflammation	IIa
Therapy via antiarrhythmic medications can be useful in patients with ventricular arrhythmias refractory to immunosuppression therapy	IIa
Ablation with catheter can be useful in patients with cardiac sarcoidosis and ventricular arrhythmias refractory to immunosuppression and antiarrhythmic therapy	IIa
Indications for implantable cardioverter	
Spontaneous sustained ventricular arrhythmias, including previous cardiac arrest	I
Ejection fraction of the left ventricle smaller or equal to 35% even with optimal medical management and a period of immunosuppression (if there was active inflammation)	I
Implantation of cardioverter can be considered in cardiac sarcoidosis independent from ventricular function in one or more of the following: • Indication of permanent pacemaker implantation • Unexplained syncope or pre-syncope, if it is of arrhythmic etiology • Inducible sustained ventricular arrhythmias	IIa
Cardioverter implantation can be considered in patients with ejection fraction from 36 to 49% and/or ejection fraction of the right ventricle below 40%, even with optimal medical management for cardiac failure and a period of immunosuppression (if there was active inflammation).	IIb
Stratification of sudden death risk	
An electrophysiological study for the stratification of sudden death can be considered in patients with ejection fraction of the left ventricle >35% even with optimal medical management for cardiac failure and a period of immunosuppression (if there was active inflammation).	IIb
Cardiac magnetic resonance imaging can be considered for the stratification of sudden death risk.	IIb

Table 4.
Management of conduction malfunctions.

9. Prognosis

In a relatively long series, Tokuda et al. [33] compared behavior and course of the cardiac sarcoidosis, after ablation with ventricular tachycardia catheter in patients with sarcoidosis and patients with other types of dilated nonischemic cardiopathies; 23% of the patients with sarcoidosis had previous arrhythmic storm, and 31% had a previous ablation and had been refactored for management with two antiarrhythmics. More than 50% had received amiodarone or beta-blockers. Although they all shared similar mechanisms of arrhythmogenesis with other types of cardiopathies, the group of patients with sarcoidosis had a higher rate of recurrence of ventricular tachycardia. After ablation, survival, or rehospitalization related to the recurrence of ventricular arrhythmias, was greater in patients with cardiac sarcoidosis. This shows that sarcoidosis has the worst prognosis among all other forms of nonischemic cardiopathy.

Author details

Jhan Carlos Altamar Castillo[1*] and Miguel Jose Tejeda Camargo[2]

1 Specialist in cardiovascular electrophysiology General Clinic of the North, Barranquilla, Colombia

2 Fellow of Cardiovascular Electrophysiology, University of La Sabana, Cardioinfantil Foundation - Institute of Cardiology, Bogota, Colombia

*Address all correspondence to: jcarlomed@gmail.com

References

[1] Okada DR, Bravo PE, Vita T, Agarwal V, Osborne MT, Taqueti VR, et al. Isolated cardiac sarcoidosis: A focused review of an under-recognized entity. Journal of Nuclear Cardiology. Aug 2018;**25**(4):1136-1146

[2] Semenzato G. ACCESS: A case control etiologic study of sarcoidosis. Sarcoidosis, Vasculitis, and Diffuse Lung Diseases. 2005;**22**(2):83-86

[3] Yatsynovich Y, Dittoe N, Petrov M, Maroz N. Cardiac sarcoidosis: A review of contemporary challenges in diagnosis and treatment. The American Journal of the Medical Sciences. 2018;**355**(2):113-125

[4] Birnie DH, Nery PB, Ha AC, Beanlands RS. Cardiac sarcoidosis. Journal of the American College of Cardiology. 2016;**68**(4):411-421

[5] Kandolin R, Lehtonen J, Airaksinen J, Vihinen T, Miettinen H, Ylitalo K, et al. Cardiac sarcoidosis: Epidemiology, characteristics, and outcome over 25 years in a nationwide study. Circulation. 2015;**131**(7):624-632

[6] Altamar Jhan A, Carlos T, Diego R, Luis S. Ventricular arrhythmias as a first sign of primary cardiac sarcoidosis. Revista Colombiana de Cardiología. 2017;**24**(5):511

[7] Patterson KC, Chen ES. The pathogenesis of pulmonary sarcoidosis and implications for treatment. Chest. 2018;**153**(6):1432-1442

[8] Sakthivel P, Bruder D. Mechanism of granuloma formation in sarcoidosis. Current Opinion in Hematology. 2017;**24**(1):59-65

[9] Nery PB, Beanlands RS, Nair GM, Green M, Yang J, McArdle BA, et al. Atrioventricular block as the initial manifestation of cardiac sarcoidosis in middle-aged adults. Journal of Cardiovascular Electrophysiology. 2014;**25**(8):875-881

[10] Viles-Gonzalez JF, Pastori L, Fischer A, Wisnivesky JP, Goldman MG, Mehta D. Supraventricular arrhythmias in patients with cardiac sarcoidosis prevalence, predictors, and clinical implications. Chest. 2013;**143**(4):1085-1090

[11] Kron J, Ellenbogen KA. Cardiac sarcoidosis: Contemporary review. Journal of Cardiovascular Electrophysiology. 2015;**26**(1):104-109

[12] Patel MB, Mor-Avi V, Murtagh G, Bonham CA, Laffin LJ, Hogarth DK, et al. Right heart involvement in patients with sarcoidosis. Echocardiography. 2016;**33**(5):734-741

[13] Kanaroglou S, Nair V, Fernandes JR. Sudden cardiac death due to coronary artery dissection as a complication of cardiac sarcoidosis. Cardiovascular Pathology. 2015;**24**(4):244-246

[14] Ward EV, Nazari J, Edelman RR. Coronary artery vasculitis as a presentation of cardiac sarcoidosis. Circulation. 2012;**125**(6):e344-e346

[15] Soejima K, Yada H. The work-up and management of patients with apparent or subclinical cardiac sarcoidosis: With emphasis on the associated heart rhythm abnormalities. Journal of Cardiovascular Electrophysiology. 2009;**20**(5):578-583

[16] Keijsers RG, Veltkamp M, Grutters JC. Chest imaging. Clinics in Chest Medicine. 2015;**36**(4):603-619

[17] Ganeshan D, Menias CO, Lubner MG, Pickhardt PJ, Sandrasegaran K, Bhalla S. Sarcoidosis

from head to toe: What the radiologist needs to know. Radiographics. 2018;**38**(4):1180-1200

[18] Hamzeh N, Steckman DA, Sauer WH, Judson MA. Pathophysiology and clinical management of cardiac sarcoidosis. Nature Reviews. Cardiology. 2015;**12**(5):278-288

[19] Zipse MM, Sauer WH. Electrophysiologic manifestations of cardiac sarcoidosis. Current Opinion in Pulmonary Medicine. 2013;**19**(5):485-492

[20] Freeman AM, Curran-Everett D, Weinberger HD, Fenster BE, Buckner JK, Gottschall EB, et al. Predictors of cardiac sarcoidosis using commonly available cardiac studies. The American Journal of Cardiology. 2013;**112**(2):280-285

[21] Pizarro C, Kluenker F, Hammerstingl C, Skowasch D. Diagnostic value of speckle-tracking echocardiography in confirmed cardiac sarcoidosis. Clinical Research in Cardiology. 2016;**105**(10):884-886

[22] Vignaux O, Dhote R, Duboc D, Blanche P, Dusser D, Weber S, et al. Clinical significance of myocardial magnetic resonance abnormalities in patients with sarcoidosis: A 1-year follow-up study. Chest. 2002;**122**(6):1895-1901

[23] Smedema JP, Snoep G, van Kroonenburgh MP, van Geuns RJ, Dassen WR, Gorgels AP, et al. Evaluation of the accuracy of gadolinium-enhanced cardiovascular magnetic resonance in the diagnosis of cardiac sarcoidosis. Journal of the American College of Cardiology. 2005;**45**(10):1683-1690

[24] Ichinose A, Otani H, Oikawa M, Takase K, Saito H, Shimokawa H, et al. MRI of cardiac sarcoidosis: Basal and subepicardial localization of myocardial lesions and their effect on left ventricular function. AJR. American Journal of Roentgenology. 2008;**191**(3):862-869

[25] Tadamura E, Yamamuro M, Kubo S, Kanao S, Hosokawa R, Kimura T, et al. Images in cardiovascular medicine. Multimodality imaging of cardiac sarcoidosis before and after steroid therapy. Circulation. 2006;**113**(20):e771-e773

[26] Youssef G, Leung E, Mylonas I, Nery P, Williams K, Wisenberg G, et al. The use of 18F-FDG PET in the diagnosis of cardiac sarcoidosis: A systematic review and meta analysis including the Ontario experience. Journal of Nuclear Medicine. 2012;**53**(2):241-248

[27] Birnie DH, Sauer WH, Bogun F, Cooper JM, Culver DA, Duvernoy CS, et al. HRS expert consensus statement on the diagnosis and management of arrhythmias associated with cardiac sarcoidosis. Heart Rhythm. 2014;**11**(7):1305-1323

[28] Gungor S, Ozseker F, Yalcinsoy M, Akkaya E, Can G, Eroglu H, et al. Conventional markers in determination of activity of sarcoidosis. International Immunopharmacology. 2015;**25**(1):174-179

[29] Bennett MK, Gilotra NA, Harrington C, Rao S, Dunn JM, Freitag TB, et al. Evaluation of the role of endomyocardial biopsy in 851 patients with unexplained heart failure from 2000-2009. Circulation. Heart Failure. 2013;**6**(4):676-684

[30] Liang JJ, Hebl VB, DeSimone CV, Madhavan M, Nanda S, Kapa S, et al. Electrogram guidance: A method to increase the precision and diagnostic yield of endomyocardial biopsy for suspected cardiac sarcoidosis and myocarditis. JACC: Heart Failure. 2014;**2**(5):466-473

[31] Vaidya VR, Abudan AA, Vasudevan K, Shantha G, Cooper LT, Kapa S, et al. The efficacy and safety of electroanatomic mapping-guided endomyocardial biopsy: A systematic review. Journal of Interventional Cardiac Electrophysiology. 2018

[32] Yazaki Y, Isobe M, Hiroe M, Morimoto S, Hiramitsu S, Nakano T, et al. Prognostic determinants of long-term survival in Japanese patients with cardiac sarcoidosis treated with prednisone. The American Journal of Cardiology. 2001;**88**(9):1006-1010

[33] Tokuda M, Tedrow UB, Kojodjojo P, Inada K, Koplan BA, Michaud GF, et al. Catheter ablation of ventricular tachycardia in nonischemic heart disease. Circulation. Arrhythmia and Electrophysiology. 2012;**5**(5):992-1000

Chapter 8

Particularities of Hepatic Sarcoidosis

Laura Iliescu and Letitia Toma

Abstract

Liver sarcoidosis is usually an underdiagnosed disease, which can have severe implications in the evolution of a patient. Due to the fact that sarcoidosis is a disease based on immunological disorders, it is only natural that the liver should be one of the first organs to be affected. The imaging of liver sarcoidosis is of marked importance, especially in the differential diagnosis of the disease. While the histology aspect of sarcoidosis is relatively clear and should prompt a positive diagnosis, finding a liver granuloma in ultrasonography raises a multitude of questions and implies extensive testing for diagnosis. Furthermore, treatment of liver sarcoidosis is controversial, taking into account the possibility of developing end-stage liver disease in patients with a long history of sarcoidosis. This chapter aims to review diagnostic and treatment options for liver sarcoidosis and to determine the best management of these patients.

Keywords: liver granuloma, sarcoidosis, cholestasis, abdominal ultrasonography, liver transplant

1. Introduction

Liver granulomas may appear as either a primary condition or secondary to systemic disease [1]. They consist of modified macrophages and other inflammatory cells that adhere due to antigenic stimulation. If there is liver inflammation within or surrounding these granulomas, the term used is granulomatous hepatitis.

The prevalence of liver granulomas is as high as 15% in biopsy specimens in the general population [2], with a higher frequency (up to 75%) in special populations like HIV-infected patients and patients with prolonged fever of unknown etiology [3].

Common causes of liver granulomas include primary biliary cirrhosis, sarcoidosis, infectious diseases (*Mycobacterium tuberculosis*, Listeria, Histoplasma, Schistosoma and hepatitis C virus), drugs and malignancies [1]. However, up to 36% of all liver granulomas are of unknown etiology [4].

Granuloma formation takes place during a chronic inflammation reaction, involving epithelioid cells, lymphocytes, monocytes and plasma cells, recruited under the influence of T-cell interleukins [1]. The reaction is consistent with a delayed hypersensitivity cellular immune response to pathogenic material.

2. Etiology and histology of hepatic sarcoidosis

Sarcoidosis is a non-caseating granulomatous disease, of unknown etiology, affecting primarily mediastinum lymph nodes and the lungs. Its diagnosis is mainly an exclusion one, requiring elimination of all infectious and antigen-producing diseases [5]. The pathognomonic histological aspect is of non-caseating granulomas containing epithelioid cells [6]. Typically, sarcoidosis affects the lungs in over 90% of the cases, but several other organs may be involved, including the liver, the skin, the central nervous system, the heart and the eyes [7, 8]. The main peak of incidence is described for the age group 20–39 years for both genders, with women having a second incidence peak at the ages of 65–69 [9].

The main pathophysiological process in sarcoidosis is the immune paradox, with exaggerated inflammation at disease sites and relative anergy in the unaffected regions [10]. Several theories have been suggested as explanation for this paradox [11]. First, there may be an imbalance between regulatory and effector T-cell lymphocytes that accumulate in the periphery of the granuloma and exert inhibiting effects on naïve T cells. Second, the intense immune stimulation at the disease sites causes lymphocytes to converge in these sites and produces a relative peripheral leukopenia. Third, subsequent to disease chronicity, immunosuppressive T cells are more abundant in the peripheral blood, producing anergy to other antigen stimulations.

The result of this immune imbalance is the non-caseous granuloma, probably containing a partially degraded antigen surrounded by macrophages and T-helper cells. [11]. These macrophages will in turn differentiate into epithelioid cells that will eventually fuse to form multinucleate giant cells. The periphery of the granuloma contains CD8+ T cells, regulatory T cells, fibroblasts and B cells.

As mentioned before, a large percentage of patients with sarcoidosis present with typical signs of the disease in liver biopsy specimens, while only 10–30% have abnormal liver tests [12]. Risk factors associated with liver involvement in sarcoidosis include African-American ethnicity, exposure to pegylated interferon and splenomegaly [13].

The histology aspect of liver sarcoidosis is defined by the presence of epithelioid granulomas in both the portal tracts and hepatic lobules [14]. About 30% of patients with liver sarcoidosis have histological chances similar to those in primary biliary cirrhosis or primary sclerosing cholangitis [15]. However, typical granulomas in sarcoidosis are larger, better defined and associated with multinucleate giant cells. Occasionally, the granulomas may conflate resulting in large masses, which can be misdiagnosed for liver tumors on abdominal imaging [15]. Furthermore, granulomas from primary biliary cirrhosis are portal based and are associated with bile duct destruction, unlike sarcoidosis. In sarcoidosis, there are other signs of organ involvement, as it is a systemic disease, and anti-mitochondrial antibodies are always negative. The histological differential diagnosis between liver sarcoidosis and drug-induced liver injury (DILI) takes into account the fact that DILI manifests as granulomatous hepatitis, with small intralobular granulomas with periportal inflammation [16].

The most important aspect of differentiation between sarcoidosis and infectious granulomas is the presence of caseous necrosis, typical for infectious granulomas [17]. As such, caseating granulomas with central necrosis must be considered infections, until serious evidence eliminates the diagnosis. However, histochemical stains have a low sensitivity for infections, and false-negative results are frequent.

The histology aspect of sarcoidosis may vary, thus explaining the differences in symptomatology and evolution [15]. In a report of 100 cases with sarcoidosis and liver biopsy due to abnormal liver test results, all patients presented with liver granulomas, 99% non-caseating, frequently located in the periportal region. None of the patients had serology or cultures suggestive for infectious granulomas. Three types of histologic alterations were encountered: most patients had cholestatic changes (58%), while 41% presented with necroinflammatory changes and 20% presented with vascular alterations. Patients with cholestasis presented with histology aspects similar to those encountered in primary biliary cirrhosis (19 patients with bile duct lesions) or primary sclerosing cholangitis (13 patients with periductal fibrosis). Biliary ductopenia was noted in 37 out of 58 patients with cholestasis. Twelve patients presented with acute cholangitis without signs of biliary obstruction. Necroinflammatory changes consisted of spotty necrosis and chronic portal inflammation, suggesting hepatitis of various etiologies (viral or drug-induced). Vascular alterations encountered in these patients were sinusoidal dilatation and nodular regenerative hyperplasia. Fibrosis was present in 21 patients overall: 13 patients with periportal fibrosis, 2 patients with bridging fibrosis and 6 patients with cirrhosis.

3. Clinical aspects of hepatic sarcoidosis

The spectrum of liver damage in sarcoidosis varies greatly from asymptomatic patients to end-stage liver disease [12]. Commonly, mild liver cytolysis can be observed (in about 30% of patients with positive biopsies for sarcoidosis) [12]. Abdominal imaging reveals hepatomegaly in less than 50% of the cases [18].

Non-specific symptoms are frequently encountered in patients with sarcoidosis, including malaise, fatigue, arthralgias and fever [19]. Symptoms suggesting liver involvement are jaundice, pruritus and abdominal pain in the upper right quadrant, due to chronic cholestasis and distension of the Glisson capsule by hepatomegaly containing granulomas [19, 20]. One report even describes fever and arthralgias in 70% of patients with liver sarcoidosis, as opposed to those without liver involvement [21].

Rarely, the chronic evolution of liver sarcoidosis can lead to portal hypertension and in a minority of cases, end-stage liver disease with the need for liver transplantation [19]. Also, few cases of association between liver sarcoidosis and Budd-Chiari syndrome have been reported [22]. In a report published in 2006 [23], out of 180 patients, 50% had altered liver function associated with sarcoidosis, while 13% of the patients had liver affection without lung sarcoidosis. Fourteen patients presented with liver cirrhosis from the diagnosis of liver involvement, while two patients developed cirrhosis in the course of the disease, despite corticoid therapy. Six patients underwent liver transplantation, and recurrence of liver sarcoidosis was reported in one patient after transplantation.

Case reports of liver sarcoidosis show either non-specific general symptomatology or altered liver enzymes at the time of diagnosis. For example, liver sarcoidosis was diagnosed in a 41-year-old patient with a known history of ocular and lung sarcoidosis for 6 years, who presented with an increase in liver enzymes during periodic follow-up [24]. Final diagnosis was based on positron emission tomography and subsequent liver biopsy.

Liver sarcoidosis may also appear in association with cutaneous sarcoidosis. In a report of 40 cases of patients with cutaneous sarcoidosis (with positive histology) monitored for a mean period of 9 years, 32 patients developed lung and thoracic lymph node disease; 1 patient developed liver sarcoidosis [25].

A recent case series of 7 patients with liver sarcoidosis found that the liver was affected in the evolution of known sarcoidosis in 2 cases, while the other 5 had liver involvement at the time of diagnosis [26]. Four patients presented with upper right quadrant abdominal pain and one patient had incidentally discovered altered liver enzymes on routine evaluation. One patient also presented with cutaneous sarcoidosis (erythematous lesions on the scalp), one patient had ocular involvement (Sicca syndrome), while one patient had both skin and ocular manifestations (uveitis and sarcoid nodules). Notably, hepatomegaly was observed in all 7 patients, with 2 patients presenting with concomitant splenomegaly. One of these patients was found to have primary Budd-Chiari syndrome.

Another case report presents the diagnosis of liver sarcoidosis in an asymptomatic 66-year-old woman with abnormal liver function test on routine evaluation [27], requiring extensive evaluation by tomography and magnetic resonance imaging and ultimately liver biopsy for diagnostic confirmation.

In rare instances, necrosis of the sarcoid granulomas may appear [28]. The case of a 37-year-old woman with sudden onset of fever and right abdominal pain is reported. Initially, the patient was treated for suspicion of intra-abdominal infection. The presence of liver and splenic lesions on abdominal CT scan prompted the need for liver biopsy, showing necrotizing granulomas negative for infection, with remission of symptoms after corticoid therapy.

Few cases of typical sarcoidosis have been described under the age of 20 years [29]. One case report [30] presents the diagnosis of pediatric-onset adult sarcoidosis, with lung, liver and lymph nodes involvement. The 9-year-old patient presented with asthenia, weight loss, hepatosplenomegaly and 2 palpable lymph nodes (supraclavicular and inguinal). The major aspect of this case is the emphasis on the differential diagnosis from lymphoproliferative diseases in patients with abdominal organomegaly.

Furthermore, liver sarcoidosis may evolve silently with the development of cirrhosis and portal hypertension. Such a case was reported in 2012 [31] in a 48-year-old patient, complaining of abdominal pain. CT scan in this patient revealed hepatosplenomegaly and increased diameter of portal and splenic vein, suggestive of portal hypertension. In the absence of autoimmune and viral markers, the patient underwent liver biopsy with a positive diagnosis of liver sarcoidosis. Repeated thorax CT scans did not reveal pulmonary or lymph nodes involvement. Splenectomy was required due to severe pancytopenia. The patient's evolution was complicated with the development of ascites; the authors note the absence of esophageal or gastric varices as a sign of portal hypertension in this patient.

A review of 37 patients with sarcoidosis and portal hypertension [20] found a predominance of female patients. All patients presented with hepatosplenomegaly and esophageal varices in different degrees. Direct measurement of pressure in the portal vein was performed in 18 patients, with an average portal pressure of 24.6 mmHg. The authors emphasize the different physiopathological aspects of portal hypertension in sarcoidosis: healing fibrosis, large sarcoid granulomas and small perigranular arteriovenous shunts may increase sinusoidal resistance leading to portal hypertension. A presinusoidal blockage may occur by the direct pressure of the sarcoid granulomas in the portal areas. Another possible explanation is ischemia-induced fibrosis and cirrhosis in the setting of primary granulomatous phlebitis of the portal and hepatic veins [32].

Liver sarcoidosis can be associated with chronic cholestasis, either intrahepatic (mimicking primary biliary cirrhosis or primary sclerosing cholangitis) or extrahepatic (by hilar or ductal compression by adenopathies) [20]. Clinical manifestations of intrahepatic cholestasis reported in 31 patients were pruritus, jaundice and right quadrant abdominal pain. Extrahepatic cholestasis is far rarer [33], and CT scan and endoscopic retrograde cholangiopancreatography are required for the diagnosis.

Acute sarcoidosis rarely presents with liver involvement [20]. Usually, the clinical presentation is dominated by pulmonary symptoms (cough, dyspnea and

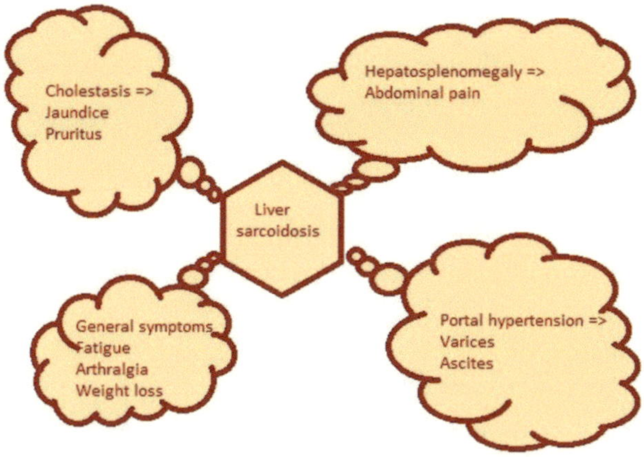

Figure 1.
Summary of clinical aspects encountered in liver sarcoidosis.

chest discomfort) and constitutional symptoms (fever, fatigue, malaise and weight loss). Liver involvement may be suspected in the presence of jaundice, pruritus or abnormal liver function tests.

Figure 1 summarizes possible clinical aspects of liver sarcoidosis.

4. Laboratory findings in liver sarcoidosis

Both cholestasis and hepatocytolysis can appear in liver sarcoidosis. Abnormal liver tests are found in up to 40% of patients with sarcoidosis, with a predominance of cholestasis (increased alkaline phosphatase (ALP), gamma-glutamyl transpeptidase (γGT) and minor increases in bilirubin levels) [34]. ALP can be increased in up to 90% of the patients with symptoms of hepatic disease, up to 10 times the upper normal limit [19]; by contrast, increases in transaminases are mild and less frequent. The severity of the cholestasis is associated with the degree of granulomatous inflammation [35].

Peripheral lymphopenia, especially noted in CD4+ positive cells, can be useful in suspecting sarcoidosis [31]. Hypercalcemia and hypercalciuria can also be found, but unrelated to liver involvement.

In cases with portal hypertension, frequent findings are pancytopenia [20, 31] with the predominance of thrombocytopenia. Hypoalbuminemia can also be encountered as a sign of liver disease.

Most laboratory determinations are aimed at excluding other causes of liver disease. Most commonly used are viral serology markers for hepatitis B and C infection, serum markers for Wilson's disease and hemochromatosis (especially in young patients), autoantibody determinations for celiac disease, primary biliary cirrhosis and autoimmune hepatitis. **Table 1** summarizes the main serum determinations to exclude other etiologies of liver disease [36].

Patients with active disease may present with increased levels of serum inflammation markers (such as erythrocyte sedimentation rate and C-reactive protein), regardless of the organs involved [37]. CRP may also be associated with fatigue in sarcoidosis. However, these tests are not specific in any way to sarcoidosis.

There are yet no serum markers for the clear diagnosis of sarcoidosis. High serum levels of angiotensin-converting enzyme have been associated with sarcoidosis and are present in about 60% of patients with active disease [19]. Nevertheless, the test is far from pathognomonic, with low positive and negative predicting values

Determination	Result	Diagnosis	Comments
HBs antigen	Positive	Hepatitis B infection	Determine HBV-DNA Search for HDV co-infection
HCV antibodies	Positive	Possible hepatitis C infection	Confirm infection with HCV- RNA
IgM antibodies for cytomegalovirus	Positive	Possible CMV hepatitis	Determine viremia
Ceruloplasmin	Low values	Possible Wilson's disease	Confirm with genetic testing
Serum copper	High values		
Urinary copper	High values		
Serum ferritin	High values	Possible hemochromatosis	Confirm with genetic testing/liver biopsy
Transferrin levels	High values		
Antinuclear antibodies	Positive	Possible autoimmune hepatitis	Search for concurrent abnormal tests and/or other organ involved
Antismooth muscle antibodies (SMA)	Positive	Possible autoimmune hepatitis	
Antiliver kidney muscle antibodies (LKM-1)	Positive	Possible autoimmune hepatitis	
Antimitochondrial antibodies	Positive	Possible primary biliary cirrhosis	
Antineutrophil cytoplasmic antibodies	Positive	Possible Wegener's disease, other vasculitis	
Anti-*Saccharomyces cerevisiae*	Positive	Possible inflammatory bowel disease, associated with primary biliary cirrhosis	
Antitissue transglutaminase	Positive	Possible celiac disease	

Table 1.
Biological parameters required in the etiology of liver disease (adapted from [36]).

(84% and 74%, respectively). Normal ACE levels should not be used for exclusion of sarcoidosis-they can be encountered in patients with chronic disease or patients under corticoid therapy. High values are indicative of sarcoidosis and can be used in excluding other granulomatous diseases. However, inflammatory bowel disease can also manifest with high level of ACE, and the differential diagnosis is difficult, especially when primary biliary cirrhosis is associated. Increased levels of ACE can also be found in pulmonary silicosis, asbestosis, military tuberculosis, diabetes mellitus and hyperthyroidism [38].

5. Imaging in liver sarcoidosis

In asymptomatic patients, a routine laboratory testing or abdominal ultrasound can raise suspicion of liver disease, especially in the setting of a known history of sarcoidosis. In fact, some authors recommend routine testing for liver sarcoidosis in the course of the disease [19].

Abdominal ultrasonography frequently reveals hepatomegaly, possibly associated with splenomegaly in the case of splenic involvement or portal hypertension. One review found that 8% of patients with liver sarcoidosis had marked hepatomegaly, with an anteroposterior diameter of over 25 cm [39]. The general aspect of the liver is of increased echogenicity, either homogenous or diffusely heterogeneous [40] (**Figure 2**). The aspect sometimes may resemble fatty liver disease [41].

Focal liver nodules may appear on ultrasonography in the case when sarcoid granulomas conflate and form macroscopic masses. Such nodules have been described in up to 19% of patients [40]. Typically, there are innumerous round nodules, diffusely distributed, with size ranging from 1 to 2 mm to centimeters [39]. Color Doppler ultrasonography reveals hypovascularization of the nodules.

Splenomegaly is also reported in almost 60% of patients with liver sarcoidosis [40], with markedly increased dimensions (over 18 cm) in 6% of the cases. In 15% of cases, splenomegaly is associated with hypoechoic splenic nodules. The frequency of nodules appears to vary according to geographical distribution and ethnic characteristics [40]. They are distributed diffusely within the splenic parenchyma, with a medium size of 1 cm [42]; they demonstrate hypovascularization on Doppler analysis. Isolated splenic nodules are more frequent than isolated hepatomegaly or liver nodules in sarcoidosis.

Up to 76% of patients with liver and splenic nodules also associate with enlarged abdominal lymph nodes [43], with infrequent punctate calcifications. Adenopathies are usually found periportal, celiac, paracaval and para-aortic, with dimensions ranging from 1 cm to 4–6 cm [44, 45]. Larger perihepatic lymph nodes can be associated with advanced liver disease. They raise the need for differential diagnosis to malignant conditions (primarily lymphoproliferative disorders), intra-abdominal infections and benign conditions such as primary biliary cirrhosis or chronic hepatitis C.

Contrast-enhanced ultrasonography (CEUS) has emerged as a new, reliable and non-invasive means of evaluation of liver disease [45]. CEUS has proven its greatest utility in differentiating between benign and malignant liver and splenic nodules, with sensitivity and specificity similar to those of CT scans. The use of CEUS in abdominal sarcoidosis has been evaluated in small case series or case reports [45], due to the scarcity of the cases and also to the fact that patients with hepatosplenic sarcoidosis rarely present with focal lesions, making them difficult candidates for CEUS (**Figure 3**).

If hypoechoic liver lesions appear on conventional ultrasonography, they have variable arterial enhancement with progressive washout in the portal and late phases [45].

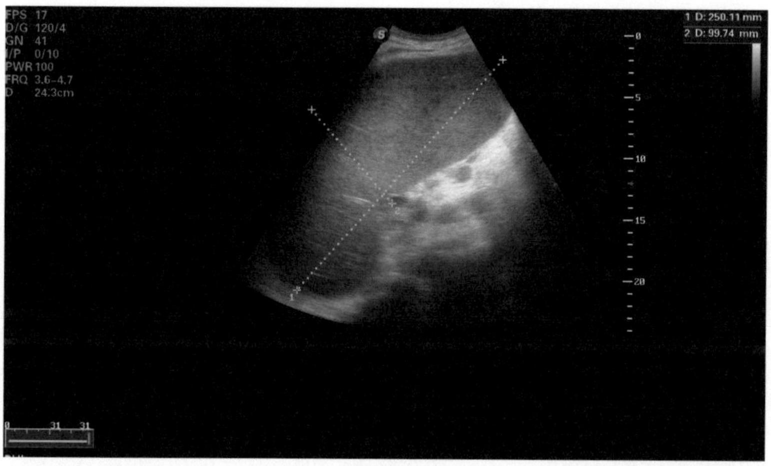

Figure 2.
Abdominal ultrasonography revealing diffusely heterogeneous hepatomegaly in a patient with liver sarcoidosis.

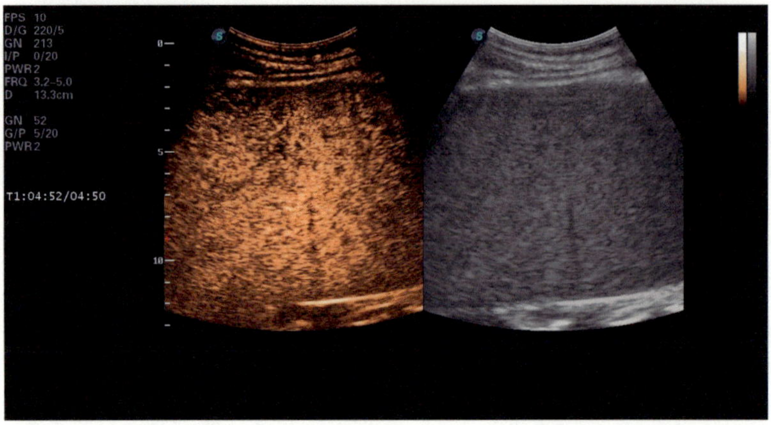

Figure 3.
CEUS in a patient with liver sarcoidosis—diffuse disease, without focal lesions (late phase).

Regarding hypoechoic splenic nodules, on CEUS, they appear as progressive hypoenhancing nodules in the arterial and parenchymal phases. As the investigation progresses into the parenchymal phase, the lesion-to-parenchyma contrast diffusion is increased. The mild enhancement in the arterial phase can be homogenous or diffusely heterogeneous, while in the parenchymal phase, it may be homogenous or with a dotted pattern. Sometimes, peripheral blood vessels may be visible and have an irregular aspect. These characteristics may be compatible with malignant conditions; therefore, biopsy is mandatory for a clear diagnosis.

A study performed in 2013 evaluated the efficacy of CEUS in diagnostic abdominal disease in 21 patients with pulmonary sarcoidosis [46]. Eighteen patients had no hepatosplenic disease, one patient had splenic nodules and two patients had liver lesions. CEUS as well as CT scan and abdominal MRI gave concordant results. The authors underline the importance of CEUS in the evaluation of these patients, as it offers the same information without any contraindications that CT or MRI might have including allergy to contrast, contrast-induced nephropathy or the presence of pacemakers or metallic devices. It is also suggested that CEUS should be used in the first evaluation of patients with pulmonary sarcoidosis and in their monitorization during treatment.

The latest review on the importance of CEUS in the evaluation of abdominal involvement in sarcoidosis describes the following characteristics [47]:

- Liver aspect on CEUS: variable nodular enhancement in the arterial phase, progressive hypoenhancement in the portal and late phases.

- Splenic aspect on CEUS: progressive hypoenhancement in the arterial and parenchymal phase. Possible patterns: rim-like, homogenous, dotted.

Endoscopic ultrasound elastography could also be used to characterize liver sarcoidosis [47]. The lesions may appear as single masses with blue hard patterns within and around.

However, the lack of sufficient data especially from clinical trials or large studies makes it impossible to establish clear recommendations on the use of CEUS in liver sarcoidosis; therefore, other imagistic methods are required for a complete positive diagnosis.

CT scans in liver sarcoidosis may reveal homogenous hepatomegaly (with possible low-density intrahepatic septa) [40] (**Figure 4**). Liver nodules appear as hypoenhanced masses as opposed to the adjacent normal liver parenchyma. There is

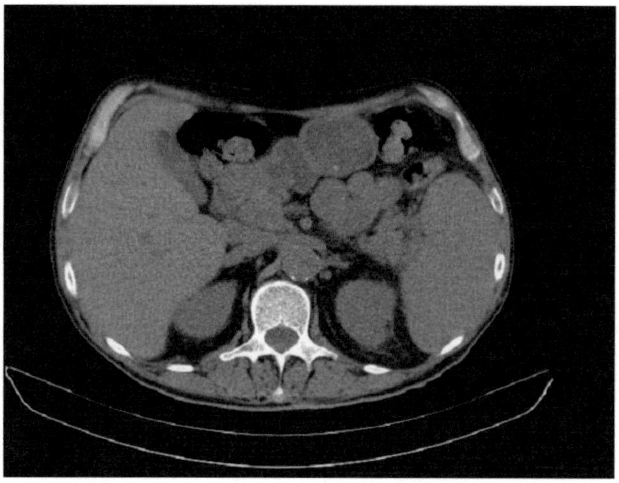

Figure 4.
Abdominal CT scan of a patient with liver sarcoidosis showing homogeneous hepatomegaly and splenomegaly.

no visible peripheral enhancement. Typically, the nodules have no mass effect. Sometimes, these numerous hypodense nodules with variable dimensions warrant differential diagnosis to metastatic disease of the liver, but also miliary liver tuberculosis, fungal infections or Langerhans cell histiocytosis [48].

CT scan is useful in the diagnosis of liver cirrhosis and portal hypertension subsequent to sarcoidosis [49], as rare as they appear. Typical aspects include hypertrophy of the caudate lobe, dilatation of the portal and splenic veins, irregular liver contour, collateral circulation vessels around the digestive tract as well as ascites.

MRI evaluation of liver sarcoidosis may reveal hypointense and hypoenhancing nodules relative to the adjacent liver parenchyma [40] (**Figures 5** and **6**). Still, the particularity of the imaging is the lack of mass effect or any impact of the nodules on the surrounding parenchyma or adjacent vessels.

T2-weighted fat-saturated images are the most conclusive in diagnosing hypointense nodules in liver sarcoidosis. This is an important part in the differential diagnosis from malignancies, as these appear most frequently as hyperintense. Other signs suggestive of sarcoidosis are irregular contour of the liver and high periportal

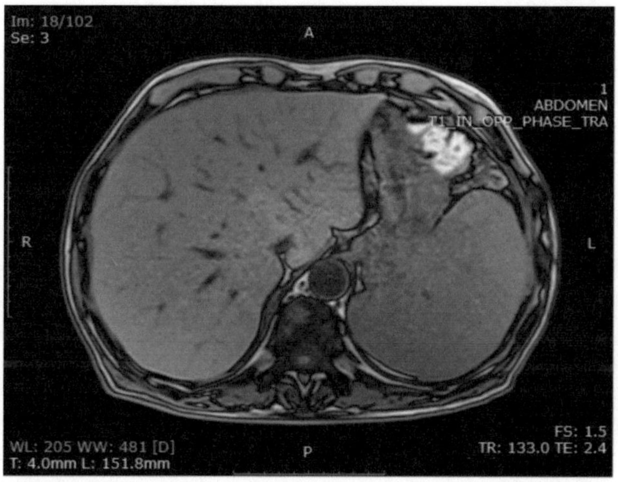

Figure 5.
MRI of a patient with diffuse liver sarcoidosis.

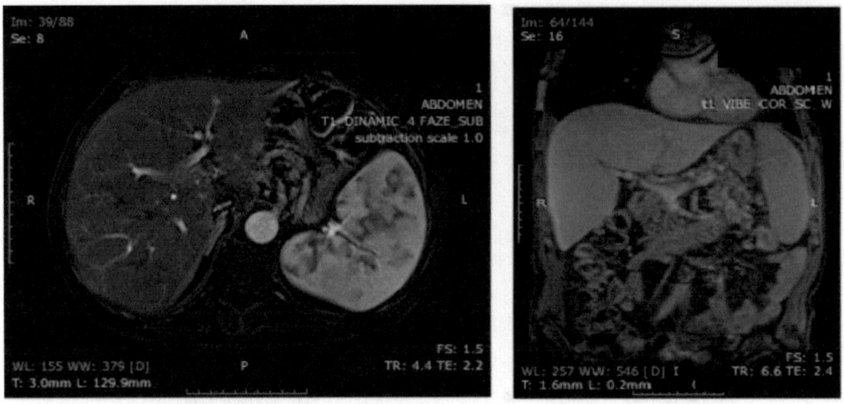

A B

Figure 6.
MRI in a patient with liver and splenic sarcoidosis demonstrating hypoattenuation of splenic lesions (A). MRI in the same patient demonstrating hepatosplenomegaly (B).

signal intensity [50]. However, cases have been described where masses with T2 hyperintensity have proven to be liver sarcoidosis in histology examination [51].

Nodules located in the hilar area need to be differentiated from cholangiocarcinomas. In cases thus located or in the case of hilum adenopathies and subsequent stenosis of biliary ducts, magnetic resonance cholangiopancreatography may reveal the stenosis with dilatation of intrahepatic bile ducts, similar to that in a Klatskin tumor [52]. In this case, the positive diagnosis is set by biopsy, usually obtained by ERCP.

6. Management of liver sarcoidosis

Guidelines for the management of sarcoidosis are relatively old and have little approach to the possibility of liver sarcoidosis [53]. Staging of sarcoidosis takes into account the pulmonary and mediastinal lymph node involvement, without considering systemic disease. Recommendations for monitoring are as follows:

- Surveillance for 2 years to determine the need for systemic therapy (taking into account the fact that many patients present spontaneous remission).

- Therapy should be initiated in patients with severe, active or progressive disease.

- Patients with remission after corticoid therapy should be more closely monitored as the relapse rate is higher than in patients with spontaneous remission.

Mild disease (including skin lesions, uveitis and respiratory symptoms) may be managed with topical steroids. Systemic or progressive disease can be managed with systemic corticotherapy, and if necessary cytotoxic therapy or antimalaric agents. Cardiac or neurologic involvement, hypercalcemia and ocular disease not responsive to topic therapy are clear indications for systemic therapy. Regarding pulmonary disease, the consensus is that progressive pulmonary infiltrates or progressive decrease in pulmonary function may require medical therapy. Recent reviews [5, 54] support the idea of initiating therapy in the case of systemic disease with potential of progression to permanent organ damage or life-threatening conditions (such as arrhythmias).

Data for the management of liver sarcoidosis is gathered from small trials and case reports. The following recommendations may be followed:

- In patients with asymptomatic liver disease or mildly elevated liver enzymes without cholestasis, observation is required. Incidentally discovered hepatomegaly falls under this category [55].

- In patients with symptomatic liver disease, cholestasis or risk for hepatic complications, medical treatment is required.

The first line of treatment includes steroids and ursodeoxycholic acid (UDCA). Alternatively, azathioprine, methotrexate, glutathione, cyclosporine, cyclophosphamide, thalidomide and infliximab have been studied in the management of liver sarcoidosis.

The beneficial effect of corticosteroids is based on their ability to suppress the inflammatory response, thus decreasing the number of liver granulomas and the liver size, as well as ameliorating constitutional symptoms. Low-dose prednisone (10–20 mg/day) is recommended for patients with mild disease, while higher doses can be required in patients with severe symptoms. Treatment duration varies according to clinical and laboratory response, with up to 1 year of treatment before tapering the doses [56]. However, steroids have not proven beneficial for asymptomatic patients or patients with advanced stages of liver disease, including cirrhosis and portal hypertension [19].

UDCA has proven effective especially in patients with liver sarcoidosis manifested by pruritus. Recent trials has also proven its effect on delaying disease progression. One study has even proved that UDCA is superior to prednisone in improving cytolysis syndrome, pruritus and fatigue [57]. The usual daily dose of UDCA is 13–15 mg/kg.

Table 2 summarizes case reports with unusual treatment and evolution of liver sarcoidosis.

Drug	Dosage	Time to improvement	Remarks	Reference
Infliximab	3 mg/kg at 8 weeks	6 weeks	A patient with cirrhosis, portal hypertension and refractory ascites	[58]
Azathioprine	50–150 mg/kg	8 weeks	4 patients	[23]
Methotrexate	10–15 mg/week	6 months	2 patients, with improvement in liver function tests	[59]
Leflunomide	20 mg/day	6 months	1 patient	[60]
Cyclosporine	20–200 mg/day	Mean treatment duration 4 years	9 patients after liver transplantation for sarcoidosis	[61]
Thalidomide	100–200 mg/kg	7–12 months	3 patients with concomitant skin lesions	[62]
Mycophenolate mofetil	250 mg/m^2 up to 1 g/m^2	1 month	1 patient with pediatric-onset adult sarcoidosis	[30]

Table 2.
Treatment options for liver sarcoidosis.

Nevertheless, it is essential to remember standard treatment measures in patients with advanced liver disease [19]. These patients may benefit from liver transplantation, with 60% survival at 5 years [63]. Careful monitoring is required as reports of sarcoidosis recurrence after transplantation have emerged.

7. Conclusions

Liver sarcoidosis is a frequent involvement in an otherwise rare disease. Having an incompletely elucidated etiology, its clinical and biological spectrum is extremely vast, and with few reports and no substantial clinical trials, its management is mainly patient-based. However, suspicion of systemic sarcoidosis in a patient should warrant extensive evaluation for associated liver disease, as this may impact the prognosis of the patient in the clinical history. The fact that this condition can progress to end-stage liver disease and can represent an indication for liver transplantation should set sarcoidosis among hepatopathies to be clearly diagnosed and monitored.

Acknowledgements

This paper was not funded by any institution.

Conflict of interest

The authors declare no conflict of interest.

Author details

Laura Iliescu[1,2]* and Letitia Toma[1,2]

1 Fundeni Clinical Institute, Bucharest, Romania

2 "Carol Davila" University of Medicine and Pharmacy, Bucharest, Romania

*Address all correspondence to: laura_ate@yahoo.com

References

[1] Coash M, Forouhar F, Wu CH, Wu GY. Granulomatous liver diseases: A review. Journal of the Formosan Medical Association. 2012;**111**(1):3-13. DOI: 10.1016/j.jfma.2011.11.023 ISSN 0929-6646

[2] Conn HO, Klatskin G. Histopathology of Liver. London: Oxford University Press; 1993. pp. 293-311

[3] Sharma S. Granulomatous diseases of the liver. In: Zakim D, Boyer T, editors. Hepatology. 4th ed. Philadelphia, PA: Saunders, Elsevier Science; 2003. pp. 1317-1330

[4] Gaya DR, Thorburn D, Oien KA, Morris AJ, Stanley AJ. Hepatic granulomas: A 10 year single centre experience. Journal of Clinical Pathology. 2003;**56**:850-853

[5] Prasse A. The diagnosis, differential diagnosis, and treatment of sarcoidosis. Deutsches Ärzteblatt International. 2016;**113**(33-34):565-574. DOI: 10.3238/arztebl.2016.0565

[6] Rosen Y. Pathology of sarcoidosis. Seminars in Respiratory and Critical Care Medicine. 2007;**28**(1):36-52

[7] Saidha S, Sotirchos ES, Eckstein C. Etiology of sarcoidosis: Does infection play a role? Yale Journal of Biology and Medicine. 2012;**85**(1):133-141

[8] Iliescu L, Herlea V, Toma L, Orban C. Association between chronic HCV hepatitis, membranoproliferative glomerulopathy and cutaneous sarcoidosis. Journal of Gastrointestinal and Liver Diseases. 2015;**24**(1):8

[9] Iannuzzi MC, Rybicki BA, Teirstein AS. Sarcoidosis. New England Journal of Medicine. 2007;**357**(21):2153-2165

[10] Miyara M, Amoura Z, Parizot C, et al. The immune paradox of sarcoidosis and regulatory T cells. Journal of Experimental Medicine. 2006;**203**(2):359-370

[11] Loke WSJ, Herbert C, Thomas PS. Sarcoidosis: Immunopathogenesis and immunological markers. International Journal of Chronic Diseases. 2013;**2013**:13, Article ID 928601

[12] Chen ESD, Moller DR. Sarcoidosis. In: Current Rheumatology Diagnosis and Treatment. 2004

[13] Judson M. Hepatic, splenic, and gastrointestinal involvement with sarcoidosis. Seminars in Respiratory and Critical Care Medicine. 2002;**23**(6):529-541

[14] Lewis J. Histopathology of granulomatous liver disease. Clinical Liver Disease. 2018;**11**(3):77-80

[15] Devaney K, Goodman Z, Epstein M, et al. Hepatic sarcoidosis. Clinicopathologic features in 100 patients. The American Journal of Surgical Pathology. 1993;**17**:1272-1280

[16] Andrade R, Lucena I, Fernandez M, et al. Drug-induced liver injury: An analysis of 461 incidences submitted to the Spanish registry over a 10-year period. Gastroenterology. 2005;**129**:512-521

[17] Lamps L. Hepatic granulomas. A review with emphasis on infectious cause. Archives of Pathology & Laboratory Medicine. 2015;**139**:867-875

[18] Ebert EC, Kierson M, Hagspiel KD. Gastrointestinal and hepatic manifestations of sarcoidosis. The American Journal of Gastroenterology. 2008;**103**:3184-3192

[19] Tadros M, Forouhar F, Wu GY. Hepatic sarcoidosis. Journal of Clinical

and Translational Hepatology. 2013;**1**(2):87-93. DOI: 10.14218/JCTH.2013.00016

[20] Blich M, Edoute Y. Clinical manifestations of sarcoid liver disease. Journal of Gastroenterology and Hepatology. 2004;**19**:732-737

[21] Hercules HD, Bethlem NM. Value of liver biopsy in sarcoidosis. Archives of Pathology & Laboratory Medicine. 1984;**108**:831-834

[22] Deniz K, Ward SC, Rosen A, Grewal P, Xu R. Budd-Chiari syndrome in sarcoidosis involving liver. Liver International. 2008;**28**:580-581

[23] Kennedy PTF, Zakaria N, Modawi SB, Papadopoulou AM, Murray-Lyon I, Du Bois RM, et al. Natural history of hepatic sarcoidosis and its response to treatment. European Journal of Gastroenterology & Hepatology. 2006;**18**:721-726

[24] Watanabe T, Jodo S. Hepatic sarcoidosis. CMAJ. 2018;**190**(33):E988. DOI: 10.1503/cmaj.180276

[25] García-Colmenero L, Sánchez-Schmidt JM, Barranco C, Pujol RM. The natural history of cutaneous sarcoidosis. Clinical spectrum and histological analysis of 40 cases. International Journal of Dermatology. 2019;**58**:178-184. DOI: 10.1111/ijd.14218

[26] Ennaifer R, Ayadi S, Romdhane H, et al. Hepatic sarcoidosis: A case series. The Pan African Medical Journal. 2016;**24**:209. DOI: 10.11604/pamj.2016.24.209.7980

[27] Giovinale M, Fonnesu C, Soriano A, et al. Atypical sarcoidosis: Case reports and review of the literature. European Review for Medical and Pharmacological Sciences. 2009;**13**(Suppl 1):37-44

[28] Abid H, Siddiqui N. A rare case of necrotizing sarcoid granulomatosis involving liver. Cureus. 2019;**11**(8):e5366. DOI: 10.7759/cureus.5366

[29] Hafner R, Vogel P. Sarcoidosis of early onset. A challenge for the pediatric rheumatologist. Clinical and Experimental Rheumatology. 1993;**11**(6):685-691

[30] Giovannini M, Luzzati M, Ferrara G, et al. Common symptoms for a rare disease in a girl with sarcoidosis: A case report. Italian Journal of Pediatrics. 2018;**44**:74. DOI: 10.1186/s13052-018-0517-6

[31] Tan CB, Rashid S, Rajan D, Gebre W, Mustacchia P. Hepatic sarcoidosis presenting as portal hypertension and liver cirrhosis: Case report and review of the literature. Case Reports in Gastroenterology. 2012;**6**:183-189. DOI: 10.1159/000338355

[32] Moreno-Merlo F, Wanless IR, Shimamatsu K, Sherman M, Greig P, Chiasson D. The role of granulomatous phlebitis and thrombosis in the pathogenesis of cirrhosis and portal hypertension in sarcoidosis. Hepatology. 1997;**26**:554-560

[33] Rezeig MA, Fashir BM. Biliary tract obstruction due to sarcoidosis: A case report. The American Journal of Gastroenterology. 1996;**92**:527-528

[34] Karagiannidis A, Karavalaki M, Koulaouzidis A. Hepatic sarcoidosis. Annals of Hepatology. 2006;**5**(4):251-256

[35] Cremers J, Drent M, Driessen A, Nieman F, Wijnen P, Baughman R, et al. Liver-test abnormalities in sarcoidosis. European Journal of Gastroenterology & Hepatology. 2012;**24**:17-24

[36] Himoto T, Nishioka M. Autoantibodies in liver disease: important clues for the diagnosis, disease activity and prognosis. Autoimmunity Highlights.

2013;**4**(2):39-53. DOI: 10.1007/s13317-013-0046-7

[37] Rothkrantz-Kos S, van Dieijen-Visser MP, Mulder PG, Drent M. Potential usefulness of inflammatory markers to monitor respiratory functional impairment in sarcoidosis. Clinical Chemistry. 2003;**49**(9):1510-1517

[38] Ahmadzai H, Thomas PS, Wakefield D. Chapter 9. Laboratory investigations and immunological testing in sarcoidosis. In: Eishi Y, editor. Sarcoidosis. Croatia: IntechOpen; 2013

[39] Warshauer DM, Dumbleton SA, Molina PL, Yankaskas BC, Parker LA, Woosley JT. Abdominal CT findings in sarcoidosis: Radiologic and clinical correlation. Radiology. 1994;**192**:93-98. DOI: 10.2214/ajr.182.1.1820015

[40] Warshauer DM, Lee JKT. Imaging manifestations of abdominal sarcoidosis. American Journal of Roentgenology. 2004;**182**(1):15-28

[41] Sartori S, Galeotti R, Calia N, Gualandi M, Nielsen I, Trevisani L, et al. Sonographically guided biopsy and sonographic monitoring in the diagnosis and follow-up of 2 cases of sarcoidosis with hepatic nodules and inconclusive thoracic findings. Journal of Ultrasound in Medicine. 2002;**21**(9):1035-1039

[42] Scott GC, Berman JL, Higgins JL Jr. CT patterns of nodular hepatic and splenic sarcoidosis: A review of the literature. Journal of Computer Assisted Tomography. 1997;**21**(3):369-372

[43] Warshauer DM, Molina PL, Hamman SM, Koehler RE, Paulson EK, Bechtold RE, et al. Nodular sarcoidosis of the liver and spleen: Analysis of 32 cases. Radiology. 1995;**195**(3):757-762

[44] Folz SJ, Johnson CD, Swensen SJ. Abdominal manifestations of sarcoidosis in CT studies. Journal of Computer Assisted Tomography. 1995;**19**(4):573-579

[45] Tana C, Dietrich CF, Schiavone C. Hepatosplenic sarcoidosis: Contrast-enhanced ultrasound findings and implications for clinical practice. BioMed Research International. 2014;**2014**:926203. DOI: 10.1155/2014/926203

[46] Grzelak P, Augsburg Ł, Majos A, Stefańczyk L, Górski P, Piotrowski W, et al. Diagnostic potential of contrast-enhanced ultrasound (CEUS) in the assessment of spleen and liver granulomas in the course of sarcoidosis. Pneumonologia i Alergologia Polska. 2013;**81**(5):424-428

[47] Tana C, Schiavone C, Ticinesi A, et al. Ultrasound imaging of abdominal sarcoidosis: State of the art. World Journal of Clinical Cases. 2019;7(7):809-818. DOI: 10.12998/wjcc.v7.i7.809

[48] Ufuk F, Herek D. CT of hepatic sarcoidosis: Small nodular lesions simulating metastatic disease. Polish Journal of Radiology. 2015;**80**:945-954. DOI: 10.12659/PJR.893330

[49] Yeom SK, Lee CH, Cha SH, Park CM. Prediction of liver cirrhosis, using diagnostic imaging tools. World Journal of Hepatology. 2015;7(17):2069-2079. DOI: 10.4254/wjh.v7.i17.2069

[50] Kessler A, Mitchell DG, Israel HL, Goldberg BB. Hepatic and splenic sarcoidosis: Ultrasound and MR imaging. Abdominal Imaging. 1993;**18**:159-163

[51] Masuda K, Takenaga S, Morikawa K, Kano A, Ojiri H. Hepatic sarcoidosis with atypical radiological manifestations: A case report. Radiology Case Reports. 2018;**13**:936-939

[52] Suzuki K, Morise Z, Furuta S, et al. Hepatic sarcoidosis mimicking hilar cholangiocarcinoma: Case report and review of the literature. Case Reports

in Gastroenterology. 2011;**5**(1):152-158. DOI: 10.1159/000323546

[53] Statement on sarcoidosis. American Journal of Respiratory and Critical Care Medicine;**160**(2):736-755

[54] West S. Current management of sarcoidosis. I: Pulmonary, cardiac, and neurologic manifestations. Current Opinion in Rheumatology. 2018;**30**(3):243-248. DOI: 10.1097/BOR.0000000000000489

[55] Cremers JP, Drent M, Baughman RP, Wijnen PA, Koek GH. Therapeutic approach of hepatic sarcoidosis. Current Opinion in Pulmonary Medicine. 2012;**18**:472-482

[56] MacArthur KL, Forouhar F, Wu GY. Intra-abdominal complications of sarcoidosis. Journal of the Formosan Medical Association. 2010;**109**:484-492

[57] Bakker GJ, Haan YC, Maillette de Buy Wenniger LJ, Beuers U. Sarcoidosis of the liver: To treat or not to treat? The Netherlands Journal of Medicine. 2012;**70**:349-356

[58] Te HS, Campbell L, Chohan S. Infliximab therapy for hepatic and intestinal sarcoidosis. Gastroenterology & Hepatology. 2007;**3**(6):447-452

[59] Lower EE, Baughman RP. The use of low dose methotrexate in refractory sarcoidosis. The American Journal of the Medical Sciences. 1990;**299**(3):153-157

[60] Sahoo DH, Bandyopadhyay D, Xu M, Pearson K, Parambil JG, Lazar CA, et al. Effectiveness and safety of leflunomide for pulmonary and extrapulmonary sarcoidosis. The European Respiratory Journal. 2011;**38**:1145-1150

[61] Casavilla FA, Gordon R, Wright HI, Gavaler JS, Starzl TE, Van Thiel DH. Clinical course after liver transplantation in patients with sarcoidosis. Annals of Internal Medicine. 1993;**118**:865-866

[62] Nguyen YT, Dupuy A, Cordoliani F, Vignon-Pennamen MD, Lebbe C, Morel P, et al. Treatment of cutaneous sarcoidosis with thalidomide. Journal of the American Academy of Dermatology. 2004;**50**:235-241

[63] Vanatta JM, Modanlou KA, Dean AG, Nezakatgoo N, Campos L, Nair S, et al. Outcomes of orthotopic liver transplantation for hepatic sarcoidosis: An analysis of the united network for organ sharing/organ procurement and transplantation network data files for a comparative study with cholestatic liver diseases. Liver Transplantation. 2011;**17**:1027-1034

Chapter 9

Sarcoid Granulomas in Malignancy

Komal Arora, Neeraj Kaur and Jae Y. Ro

Abstract

Noncaseating epithelioid granulomas without accompanying systemic symptoms of sarcoidosis have been described in association with many primary tumors where they are designated as sarcoid-like (SL) reaction. Morphologically, this SL reaction is similar to granulomas found in systemic sarcoidosis comprising of focal accumulation of epithelioid cells and multinucleated giant cells. They can be seen either adjacent to the primary malignancy or in local draining lymph nodes. Additionally, sarcoid-like granulomas can affect other organs distant from the primary neoplasm, such as the spleen, bone marrow, and skin. This sarcoid-like reaction is thought to occur as an immunologic T-cell-mediated response to antigens expressed by the neoplastic cells or soluble tumor antigens. Whether the presence of this sarcoid-like reaction has any prognostic significance in the associated neoplasm is unclear.

Keywords: sarcoid-like granulomas, malignancy, prognosis

1. Introduction

Granulomatous inflammation is a type of chronic tissue reaction characterized histologically by accumulation of epithelioid cells and multinucleated giant cells. Sarcoidosis is a systemic granulomatous disorder of unknown etiology that affects various organs. Sarcoid-like (SL) granulomas/reactions can be seen in patients with malignant tumors without the history of systemic sarcoidosis. These reactions were first described by Wolbach in 1911 [1]. Subsequently, Herxheimer in 1917 reported sarcoidal granulomas in patients with carcinomas of breast, rectum, and cystic duct [2]. These granulomas can occur either within the primary tumor, adjacent to the primary malignancy, in local draining lymph nodes, or in organs distant from the primary malignancy such as the spleen, bone marrow, and skin. This SL reaction is thought to occur in response to antigens expressed by the neoplastic cell or soluble tumor antigens that trigger a T-cell-mediated local immune response. Other etiologies of granuloma formation in patients with malignancy are co-existing sarcoidosis, infectious etiology, and reaction to therapeutic drug or procedure. The SL granulomas have been reported to occur with an average frequency of 14% in Hodgkin lymphoma cases, 7% in non-Hodgkin lymphomas, 50% in seminomas, less than 1% in sarcomas, and 4% in various carcinomas [3, 4].

2. Histologic features

Morphologically, the granulomas of SL reaction are similar to those seen in sarcoidosis. The granulomas are comprised of central focus of epithelioid cells surrounded by a rim of lymphocytes. Both Langhans-type and foreign body-type giant cells containing asteroid body and Schaumann body inclusions have been reported [5, 6]. Usually, these granulomas are noncaseating with no central necrosis. In solid tumors such as renal cell carcinomas, the granulomas have been described in intratumoral and peritumoral location as well as in the nonneoplastic kidney and draining lymph nodes [7].

3. Pathophysiology

The granuloma formation in sarcoidosis is mediated by T-cells [8]. The granulomas in SL reactions are postulated to be a T-cell-mediated immunologic reaction to soluble tumor antigens shed by the tumor cells or released during tumor necrosis [3, 9]. In the study by Kurata et al., the authors found that the solitary granulomas in SL reactions first occur between lymph sinus and T-zone, the multiple granulomas mainly occur within T-zone, and the confluent types often occupy the whole lymph node except some residual lymphoid follicles [10]. Such a pattern suggested that the granulomas grow along the T-zone, where antigen presentation mainly occurs. Recently, some authors have also hypothesized that dendritic cells play an important role in the mechanism of T-cell activation that leads to formation of granulomas [10, 11].

SL reactions have also been reported after interferon therapy in patients with malignant melanoma and after interleukin-2 therapy for renal cell carcinoma [12, 13].

4. Prognostic significance

A dense lymphocytic infiltrate at the margins of some malignant tumors such as medullary carcinoma of the breast and colonic adenocarcinoma has been associated with an improved prognosis. This improved prognosis has been attributed to an immune-mediated cytotoxic T cell response to the tumor. Similarly, the SL reactions, which are thought to be an immune response to the tumor antigens, are expected to be associated with improved prognosis.

Currently, the prognostic significance of these SL granulomas is debatable. Some authors hypothesized that SL granulomatous reactions could play an important role in the host's defense against metastatic spread [9, 14]. Several studies have shown that the presence of granulomas in Hodgkin's disease correlated with improved survival in all stages of disease [15–17]. Similarly, SL reactions in gastric carcinoma have been reported to have a good prognosis [18]. Takeuchi et al. demonstrated that the incidence of SL reactions in the regional lymph nodes decreased as gastric cancer progressed [19]. In another study on seven cases of gastric cancer associated with SL reaction, none of the patients had any episodes of recurrence, suggesting a more favorable prognosis when compared with gastric cancer patients without a SL reaction [20].

SL reactions are relatively less common in solid tumors as compared to lymphomas. In a study by Lynch et al., the authors found that SL reaction was associated with improved prognosis in small cell carcinoma of the lung [21]. Recently, Steinfort et al. [22] studied eight patients with nonsmall cell carcinoma lung where sarcoidal granulomas were present in regional lymph nodes. The authors concluded that the presence of sarcoidal reactions within regional lymph nodes of these patients predicted a lower rate of disease recurrence after definitive surgical resection. However, an earlier study by Kamiyoshihara et al. ruled out this hypothesis in lung cancer and found the SL reactions to be of no prognostic significance [23]. Similarly Tomimaru et al. studied 22 lung carcinoma patients with SL reaction in the regional lymph nodes and found no statistically significant difference in the overall survival [24].

Few cases of breast carcinoma and colorectal carcinoma associated with a stromal granulomatous SL reaction have been reported in the literature [25–30]. The authors were not able to make a definitive comment on the prognostic significance of these SL reactions in these published reports due to limited number of cases.

Recently, we published the largest case series on SL reactions in renal cell carcinoma [7]. However, due to the limited follow-up and small number of cases, we could not conclude if these SL granulomas had any prognostic significance in renal cell carcinomas. We hypothesized that the high content of glycogen and lipid in tumor cells of clear cell and clear cell papillary renal cell carcinomas possibly triggered a granulomatous reaction, similar to that seen in seminomas.

In a recent case series published by Lashari et al., the authors reported the occurrence of granulomatous mediastinal lymphadenitis at a site remote from the location of primary gynecological malignancy without evidence of metastatic disease [31].

5. Sarcoidosis coexisting with malignancy

Sarcoidosis is associated with an increased risk for cancer development in various organs such as lung, liver, or stomach [32, 33]. Many hematologic malignancies and melanomas have also been associated with sarcoidosis. Coexistence of sarcoidosis and cancer has been associated with a diminished survival rate [34]. Sarcoidosis can present in patients before, during, or after diagnosis of malignancy [35, 36].

The association between systemic sarcoidosis and malignant lymphoma was first described by Brincker in 1986. The author used the term "Sarcoidosis-lymphoma syndrome" to describe this association [37]. It refers to development of lymphoma and other hematological malignancies after diagnosis of sarcoidosis as well as includes patients with lymphoma and hematological malignancies who subsequently develop sarcoidosis [35]. Differentiating between granulomas of systemic sarcoidosis and SL granulomas in patients with malignancy is difficult based on morphology alone. Diagnosis of systemic sarcoidosis is made in the presence of additional well-recognized clinical and radiological findings.

6. Diagnostic dilemmas

Radiologically, a SL reaction can mimic tumor recurrence/deposits in the draining lymph nodes. Hence, differentiating lymphadenopathy caused by a SL reaction and metastatic disease is very important clinically. Definitive diagnosis can be made only by histopathological examination of the lymph nodes.

Granulomas in the draining lymph nodes of malignancy can be both infectious as well as SL reaction. The center of these granulomas may sometimes have nests or isolated tumor cells. Hence, a close scrutiny of such granulomas should be performed to avoid missing metastatic disease. Immunostaining with cytokeratin may be required for recognizing these in difficult cases [38].

Knowledge of the usual tumor behavior along with correlating radiologic and histologic findings is important to avoid misdiagnosis.

Author details

Komal Arora[1], Neeraj Kaur[2] and Jae Y. Ro[3]*

1 University of Pittsburgh Medical Center Horizon Hospital, Farrell, PA, United States

2 University of Texas Health Science Center, San Antonio, TX, United States

3 Houston Methodist Hospital, United States

*Address all correspondence to: jaero@houstonmetodist.org

References

[1] Wolbach SB. A new type of cell inclusion, not parasitic, associated with disseminated granulomatous lesions. Journal of Medical Research. 1911;**24**(2):243-258

[2] Herxheimer G. Uber karzinoma und tuberkulose. Zeitschrift für Tuberkulose. 1917;**27**:251-258

[3] Brincker H. Sarcoid reactions in malignant tumours. Cancer Treatment Reviews. 1986;**13**:147-156

[4] Khurana KK, Stanley MW, Powers CN, Pitman MB. Aspiration cytology of malignant neoplasms associated with granulomas and granuloma-like features: Diagnostic dilemmas. Cancer. 1998;**84**(2):84-91

[5] Nadel EM, Ackerman LV. Lesions resembling Boeck's sarcoid in lymph nodes draining an area containing a malignant neoplasm. American Journal of Clinical Pathology. 1950;**20**(10):952-957

[6] Symmers WS. Localized Tuberculoid granulomas associated with carcinoma: Their relationship to Sarcoidosis. The American Journal of Pathology. 1951;**27**(3):493-521

[7] Arora K, Divatia MK, Truong L, Shen SS, Ayala AG, Ro JY. Sarcoid-like granulomas in renal cell carcinoma: The Houston Methodist hospital experience. Annals of Diagnostic Pathology. 2017c;**31**:62-65

[8] Crystal RG, Hunninghake GW, Gadek JE, Keogh BA, Rennard SI, Bitterman PB. The pathogenesis of sarcoidosis. In: Chretien J, Marsac J, Saltiel JC, editors. Sarcoidosis and Other Granulomatous Disorders. Paris: Pergamon Press; 1981. pp. 13-35

[9] Bässler R, Birke F. Histopathology of tumour associated sarcoid-like stromal reaction in breast cancer. An analysis of 5 cases with immunohistochemical investigations. Virchows Archiv. A, Pathological Anatomy and Histopathology. 1988;**412**(3):231-239

[10] Kurata A, Terado Y, Schulz A, Fujioka Y, Franke FE. Inflammatory cells in the formation of tumor-related sarcoid reactions. Human Pathology. 2005;**36**(5):546-554

[11] Ota M, Amakawa R, Uehira K, Ito T, Yagi Y, Oshiro A, et al. Involvement of dendritic cells in sarcoidosis. Thorax. 2004;**59**:408-413

[12] Massaguer S, Sánchez M, Castel T. Mediastinal sarcoidosis induced by high-dose alpha-2-interferon therapy in a patient with malignant melanoma. European Radiology. 2004;**14**:1716-1717

[13] Logan TF, Bensadoun ES. Increased disease activity in a patient with sarcoidosis after high dose interleukin 2 treatment for metastatic renal cancer. Thorax. 2005;**60**:610-611

[14] Pavic M, Debourdeau P, Vacelet V, Rousset H. Sarcoidosis and sarcoid reactions in cancer. La Revue de Médecine Interne. 2008;**29**:39-45

[15] O'Connell MT, Schimpff SC, Kirchner RH, Aht AR, Vicrnik PH: Epithelioid granulomas in Hodgkin disease. A l·avorable prognostic sign? Journal of the American Medical Association. 1975;**233**:886-889

[16] Sacks EL, Donaldson SS, Gordon J, Dorfman RF. Epithelioid granulomas associated with Hodgkin's disease: Clinical correlations in 55 previously untreated patients. Cancer. 1978;**41**(2):562-567

[17] Brincker H. Sarcoid reactions and sarcoidosis in Hodgkin's disease and

other malignant lymphomata. British Journal of Cancer. 1972;**26**(2):120-123

[18] Nakamura M, Mizuta E, Morioka H, Nakamura M, Isiglo K. Multiple early gastric cancer associated with sarcoid-like reaction in the regional lymph nodes. Journal of Gastroenterology. 2001;**36**(10):710-717

[19] Takeuchi H, Suchi T, Suzuki R, Sato T. Histological study of immune parameters of regional lymph nodes of gastric cancer patients. GANN Japanese Journal of Cancer Research. 1982;**73**:420-428

[20] Yamamoto T, Tateishi H, Nishimura Y, Watanabe M, Ukyo S, Miyake T, et al. A study of gastric cancer with sarcoid reaction as observed in the regional lymph node. Nippon Syokakibyo Gakkai Zasshi (Japanese Journal of Gastroenterology). 1980;**77**:1555-1561

[21] Lynch JP 3rd, Flint A, Miller DM, Fantone JC. Noncaseating pulmonary granulomas associated with small cell carcinoma of the lung. The American Journal of Medicine. 1985;**78**:691-696

[22] Steinfort DP, Tsui A, Grieve J, Hibbs ML, Anderson GP, Irving LB. Sarcoidal reactions in regional lymph nodes of patients with early stage non-small cell lung cancer predict improved disease-free survival: A pilot case-control study. Human Pathology. 2012;**43**(3):333-338

[23] Kamiyoshihara M, Hirai T, Kawashima O, Ishikawa S, Morishita Y. Sarcoid reactions in primary pulmonary carcinoma: Report of seven cases. Oncology Reports. 1998;**5**:177-180

[24] Tomimaru Y, Higashiyama M, Okami J, et al. Surgical results of lung cancer with sarcoid reaction in regional lymph nodes. Japanese Journal of Clinical Oncology. 2007;**37**:90-95

[25] Oberman HA. Invasive carcinoma of the breast with granulomatous response. American Journal of Clinical Pathology. 1987;**88**:718-721

[26] Coyne J, Haboubi NY. Micro-invasive breast carcinoma with granulomatous stromal response. Histopathology. 1992;**20**:184-185

[27] Coyne JD. Colonic carcinoma with granulomatous (sarcoid) reaction. Journal of Clinical Pathology. 2002;**55**:708-709

[28] Fujii T, Tabe Y, Yajima R, et al. Adenocarcinoma of ascending Colon associated with Sarcoid reaction in regional lymph nodes. Case Reports in Gastroenterology. 2010;**4**:118-123

[29] Nozoe T, Matsumata T, Sugimachi K. Carcinoma in villous adenoma of ascending colon associated with sarcoid reaction in the regional lymph nodes. Journal of Clinical Gastroenterology. 1999;**28**:377-379

[30] Shima T, Tanaka Y, Katsuragi K, Fujio N, Nakatani S, Kobayashi Y, et al. Sarcoid reaction in the spleen after sigmoid colon cancer resection: A case report. Surgical Case Reports. 2016;**2**(1):115

[31] Lashari BH, Asai M, Randleman G, Sack M, Patel R. Sarcoid-like mediastinal lymphadenopathy in gynecologic malignancy. Pulmonary Medicine. 14 February 2018;**2018**:5141575. DOI: 10.1155/2018/5141575. eCollection 2018

[32] Spiekermann C, Kuhlencord M, Huss S, Rudack C, Weiss D. Coexistence of sarcoidosis and metastatic lesions: A diagnostic and therapeutic dilemma. Oncology Letters. 2017;**14**(6):7643-7652

[33] Askling J, Grunewald J, Eklund A, Hillerdal G, Ekbom A. Increased risk for cancer following sarcoidosis. American Journal of Respiratory and Critical Care Medicine. 1999;**160**:1668-1672

[34] Boffetta P, Rabkin CS, Gridley G. A cohort study of cancer among

sarcoidosis patients. International Journal of Cancer. 2009;**124**:2697-2700

[35] Cohen PR, Kurzrock R. Sarcoidosis and malignancy. Clinics in Dermatology. 2007;**25**(3):326-333

[36] Sehgal S, Goyal P, Ghosh S, et al. Malignancy and granulomatosis: Causality or coincidence? Narrative systematic review. Iranian Journal of Pathology. 2014;**9**:237-244

[37] Brincker H. The sarcoidosis-lymphoma syndrome. British Journal of Cancer. 1986;**54**(3):467-473

[38] Díaz Del Arco C, Aceñero MJ. Sarcoid reaction: A rare occurrence associated to colon adenocarcinoma (case report and literature review). Journal of Gastrointestinal Oncology. 2016;**7**(4):E72-E76

Chapter 10

Sarcoid Involvement of the Mammary Gland

Patricia López Arribas, Elena Martínez Gómez and Álvaro Zapico Goñi

Abstract

Sarcoidosis is a systemic granulomatous disease of unknown cause. Mammary involvement is rare, less than 1% of all cases. In addition, it makes necessary an appropriate differential diagnosis in order to rule out malignant pathology as the main diagnosis. Therefore, it is necessary to carry out different tests as mammography, ultrasound, and histological confirmation if necessary. When the diagnosis of mammary sarcoidosis is suspected by fine needle aspiration cytology, exceptional procedures should be also considered to examine for the possibility of a coexisting carcinoma. In such cases, excisional biopsy or resection is strongly recommended. There are some cases of mammary sarcoidosis associated with breast cancer. Breast cancer may develop in patients with sarcoidosis, sarcoidosis may develop in patients with breast cancer, the two diseases may develop in tandem, or breast cancer may induce a sarcoidosis-like granulomatous response. Sarcoidosis is possibly linked to silicone gel breast implants. The silicone might cause a sarcoidlike reaction as the result of an acceleration of an already existing hypersensitivity response, resulting in mammary sarcoidosis. The management of sarcoidosis in the breast usually is an excisional biopsy. At the same time, we confirm diagnosis and the treatment is done. The prognosis of mammary sarcoidosis remains unknown.

Keywords: breast sarcoidosis, granulomatous disease, mammary gland, granuloma, breast mass

1. Introduction

Sarcoidosis is a multisystemic granulomatous disorder of unknown etiology [1]. Our understanding of the pathogenesis of sarcoidosis has advanced and provided new insights into potential causes of this disease. It is important to remember that any etiologic agent of sarcoidosis must be capable of causing the pathologic hallmark of systemic noncaseating granulomas and the heterogeneous clinical features of sarcoidosis [2]. It is caused by alteration of the cellular immune response after exposure to an environmental, occupational, or infectious hazard and can involve multiple tissues and organs, including breast tissue [3].

About 80–90% of patients present lung or hiliar lymph nodes affected. These are the most common systems involved. However, the involvement of skin, eyes, nervous system, locomotor system, lacrimal and salivary glands, heart, and kidney in sarcoidosis has also been described [1].

Sarcoid involvement of the breast parenchyma has been extremely rare in patients with sarcoidosis, less than 1% of the overall diagnosed patients. It is more common in African American, Afro-Caribbean, Swedish, and Danish individuals. It typically presents in women in their third and fourth decade of life and can often mimic breast carcinoma [4].

The descriptions of breast sarcoid vary in the literature from masses with ill-defined margins or spiculated as seen in cancer, negative imaging, or other non-specific appearances [3]. The most common presentation is a palpable breast mass. Because sarcoidosis can mimic breast cancer, it makes the differential diagnosis very difficult [3].

2. Etiology

Since sarcoidosis was first described more than a century ago, the etiologic determinants causing this disease remain uncertain. Studies suggest that genetic, host immunologic, and environmental factors interact together to cause sarcoidosis. Immunologic characteristics of sarcoidosis include noncaseating granulomas, enhanced local expression of T helper-1 (and often Th17) cytokines and chemokines, dysfunctional regulatory T-cell responses, dysregulated Toll-like receptor signaling, and oligoclonal expansion of CD4+ T cells consistent with chronic antigenic stimulation. Multiple environmental agents have been suggested to cause sarcoidosis. Studies from several groups implicate mycobacterial or propionibacterial organisms in the etiology of sarcoidosis based on tissue analyses and immunologic responses in sarcoidosis patients. Despite these studies, there is no consensus on the nature of a microbial pathogenesis of sarcoidosis. Some groups postulate sarcoidosis is caused by an active viable replicating infection, while other groups contend there is no clinical, pathologic, or microbiologic evidence for such a pathogenic mechanism [2]. The authors posit a novel hypothesis that proposes that sarcoidosis is triggered by a hyperimmune Th1 response to pathogenic microbial and tissue antigens associated with the aberrant aggregation of serum amyloid A within granulomas, which promotes progressive chronic granulomatous inflammation in the absence of ongoing infection.

3. Clinical manifestations

In the breast, the clinical presentation is a breast mass that could be isolated or multiple and unilateral or bilateral. Most of the patients do not present infectious or inflammatory symptoms. Moreover the nodules are not painful. It is very important to be alert of the possible systemic symptoms that our patient may present. Sometimes breast sarcoidosis is the first diagnosis disease, but most times, the diagnosis is already done.

4. Diagnosis

The clinical impact of sarcoidosis is directly related to the extent of granulomatous inflammation and its effect on the function of vital organs.

In each patient, the sites and the severity of granulomatous involvement throughout the body must be assessed to determine the impact of sarcoidosis on systems that most greatly affect the patient's activities and quality of life or that may lead to premature death.

In the breast, the most common symptom is a breast mass. It could be only one or multiple tumors. Therefore it is very important to make a correct differential diagnosis.

First of all, the physical examination probably discloses a non-tender, firm, and mobile lesion, with no nipple abnormalities. The patient could or not present axillary lymph nodes. But in some cases the lesions were fixed or tender, clinically resembling a carcinoma.

Then, we should perform some image techniques.

Mammography, most of the time, is the first test and usually shows a nonspecific, ill-defined mass with low density, poorly outlined with no microcalcification.

We have the same problem with ultrasound examination that does not support an unequivocal diagnosis, but we are able to point out the irregularity of the contours, hypoechoic spiculation, and nonhomogeneous internal echostructure of the nodule [5] (**Figure 1**).

The next step is the high-field system MR but always complementary to the previous ones.

Images can reveal the lesion to be a solitary signal-intensive inhomogeneous tumor with irregular contours, fast contrast enhancement, and an early "wash-out" phenomenon often observed in carcinomas or in inflammatory lesions of the breast.

After that, it is important not to forget that the imaging techniques do not offer a definitive diagnosis and we must correlate it with pathological diagnosis.

To rule out infection origin, we should perform microbiologic test as stains for fungi and acid-fast bacilli.

Biopsy of the breast demonstrates chronic granulomatous inflammatory process, with epithelioid granulomas and non-necrotizing giant cells (**Figure 2**).

Breast sarcoidosis is very uncommon; most of the times, a fine needle biopsy is not enough, so an excisional biopsy is necessary.

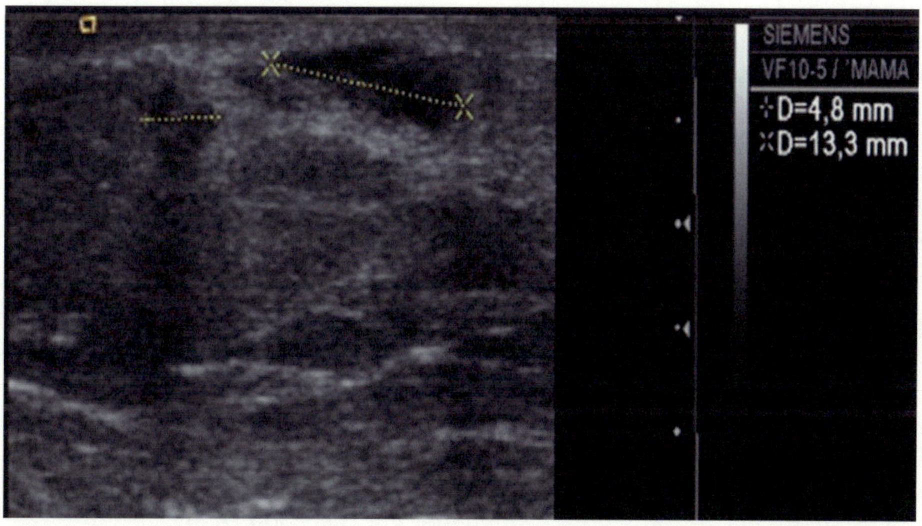

Figure 1.
Ultrasound examination with two nonspecific hypoechoic masses.

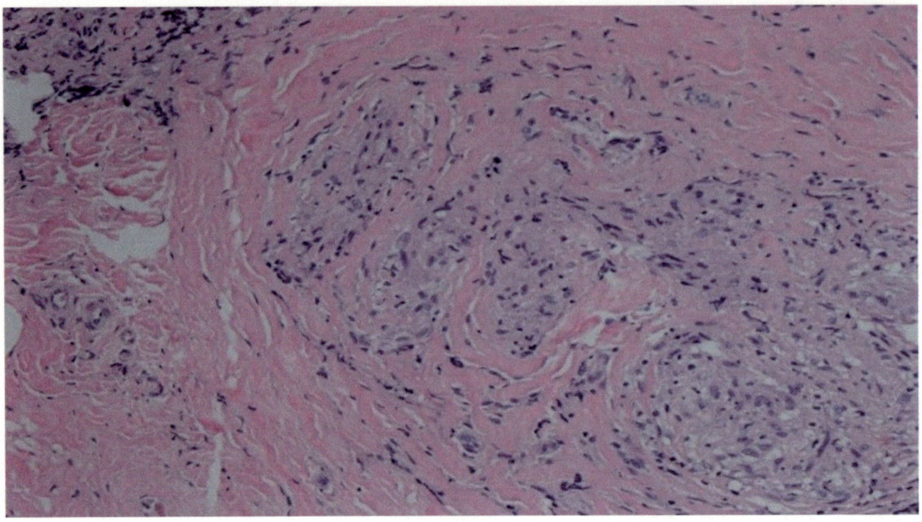

Figure 2.
Chronic granulomatous inflammatory process, with epithelioid granulomas and non-necrotizing giant cells.

The diagnosis is based on typical radiologic manifestations supported by histologic evidence of noncaseating granulomas in the absence of infection and exclusion of other types of granulomatous affections [6].

5. Differential diagnosis

There are some diseases that we should rule out when we are thinking about the diagnosis of sarcoidosis in the breast. Then, we break down each one of them.

5.1 Malignant pathology

First of all, the most important and the most frequent is malignant pathology of the breast. The American Cancer Society (ACS) estimates that 268,600 women will receive a diagnosis of invasive breast cancer and 62,930 people will receive a diagnosis of noninvasive cancer in one year. When we diagnose a breast mass, we suspect breast cancer. The initial test is mammography, ultrasound, and sometimes MRI. As we have previously objectified, there are no defined patterns in the imaging test for sarcoidosis in the breast, and we have the same problem with cancer. Therefore, we obtain a suspicious diagnosis that we need to confirm. After those techniques, we perform further tests like pathological test and immunohistochemistry to establish the definitive diagnosis, prognosis parameters, and correct therapy.

5.2 Idiopathic granulomatous mastitis (IGM)

Idiopathic granulomatous mastitis is a rare, chronic benign breast disease, which may mimic a breast abscess, malignancy, or other granulomatous pathologies. Most patients present in the third or fourth decade of life, and it typically is seen in women of childbearing potential from 6 months to 6 years postpartum. It is a diagnosis of exclusion and requires a high index of suspicion [7, 8].

Early misdiagnosis as bacterial mastitis is common, prompting multiple antibiotic regimens. When antibiotics fail, patients are worked up for inflammatory breast cancer, given the nonhealing breast nodules. Mammography, ultrasonography, and fine needle aspiration often are unable to rule out carcinoma, warranting excisional biopsies of nodules. After that, we exclude malignancy and suspect a potential sarcoidosis or IGM.

Idiopathic granulomatous mastitis is a diagnosis of exclusion, made after obtaining evidence of granulomatous inflammation on breast biopsy and ruling out other granulomatous disorders, such as tuberculosis and sarcoidosis.

Almost the totality of sarcoid patients (90%) has lung disease; when we suspect a sarcoidosis, a chest radiograph is needed to screen for hilar lymphadenopathy and sometimes an ophthalmology evaluation [8].

Many cases self-resolve, but more severe cases can persist for a long period before adequate symptomatic treatment is achieved by methotrexate, corticosteroids, or surgical excision.

5.3 Tuberculosis

Breast tuberculosis (TB) is another disease characterized by the presence of granulomas. This pathology is rare but increasingly reported in Western Europe, accounting for 4.5% of all breast lesions in TB-endemic areas and 0.1% in the developed world.

The presenting features may mimic other breast pathologies including bacterial abscess, idiopathic granulomatous mastitis, sarcoidosis, or carcinoma, making diagnosis challenging. Risk factors for the development of breast TB include immunosuppression, lactation, multiparty, and previous exposure to TB [9, 10].

The most frequent symptom is an isolated mass, with less evidence of inflammation or infection than in other types of infectious mastitis. To this, we must associate that they do not present systemic symptoms.

Diagnosis of breast TB is difficult, often necessitating multiple clinic consultations and tissue sampling procedures. This frequently results in delays in TB treatment.

5.4 Sarcoidosis-like reaction

A phenomenon known as autoimmune/inflammatory syndrome induced by adjuvants may underlie the association between silicone implants and sarcoidosis-like reaction with foreign body granulomatous reaction, in which silicone serves as an immunologic adjuvant to enhance antigen-specific immune response. This leads to enhanced production and activation of both B and T cells [11].

There are some case reports in the literature that describe this reaction, and it may take place in the breast skin, subcutaneous tissue, and also in axillary lymph nodes.

6. Treatment

The treatment of breast sarcoidosis is similar to systemic sarcoidosis, but most of the time, an excisional biopsy has to be done to confirm the diagnosis, and if the sarcoidosis is isolated in the breast, then other treatments is not necessary.

Conflict of interest

The authors declare no conflict of interest.

Author details

Patricia López Arribas*, Elena Martínez Gómez and Álvaro Zapico Goñi
Principe de Asturias University Hospital, Madrid, Spain

*Address all correspondence to: patricialopezar@gmail.com

References

[1] Takahasi R, Shibuya Y, Shijubo N, Asaishi K, Abe S. Mammary involvement in patient with sarcoidosis. Internal Medicine. 2001;**40**:769-771

[2] Chen ES, Moller DR. Etiology of sarcoidosis. Clinics in Chest Medicine. 2008;**29**:365-377

[3] Chen J, Carter R 3rd, Maoz D, Tobar A, Sharon E, Greif F. Breast cancer and sarcoidosis: Case series and review of the literature. Breast Care (Basel). 2015;**10**:137-140

[4] Nicholson BT, Mills SE. Sarcoidosis of the breast: An unusual presentation of a systemic disease. The Breast Journal. 2007;**13**:99-100

[5] Endlich JL, Souza JA, Cynthia A, Osório BT, Lopes Pinto CA, Faria EP, et al. Breast sarcoidosis as the first manifestation of the disease. Breast Journal. 2019;**00**:1-2

[6] Kenzel PP, Hadijuana J, Hosten N, Minguillon C, Oellinger H, Siewert C, et al. Boeck, sarcoidosis of the breast, ultra-sound, and MRI findings. Journal of Computer Assisted Tomography. 1997;**21**:439-441

[7] Poovamma CU, Pais VA, Dolas SC, Prema M, Khandelwal R, Nis-heena R. Idiopathic granulomatous mastitis: A rare entity with a variable presentation. Breast Disease. 2014;**34**:101

[8] Haitz K, Ly A, Smith G. Idiopathic granulomatous mastitis. Cutis. January 2019;**103**(1):38-42

[9] Mehta G, Mittal A, Verma S. Breast tuberculosis—Clinical spectrum and management. Indian Journal of Surgery. 2010;**72**(6):433-437

[10] Thimmappa D, Mallikarjuna MN, Vijayakumar A. Breast tuberculosis. Indian Journal of Surgery. 2015;**77**(3):S1378-SS138

[11] Shoenfeld Y, Agmon-Levin N. ASIA: Autoimmune/inflammatory syndrome induced by adjuvants. Journal of Autoimmunity. 2011;**36**:4-8

Chapter 11

Granulomatous Diseases Mimicking Sarcoidosis

Angel Robles-Marhuenda

Abstract

Granulomatous diseases are not infrequent in daily clinical practice. Granulomas are the expression of a sufficiently (partial) functioning immune system. Many diseases, with different etiologies (infection, autoimmunity, inflammatory, foreign bodies, malignancy, metabolites, chemicals, etc.) can cause granulomatous manifestations. The differential diagnostic process of a granulomatous disease should always be made in an interdisciplinary cooperation. Diagnostic procedures should be oriented to the clinical symptoms suggestive microbiological studies, and radiography but the diagnosis of a granulomatous disease should always be confirmed by histopathology when possible, sampling for histology or cytology. From a pathogenic point of view, they are divided into noninfectious and infectious granulomas. In the case of proven granulomatous inflammation, an infectious etiology should first be excluded (including mycobacteria, parasites, and fungi). From a clinical point of view, it is useful to separate granulomatosis into localized and disseminated forms, although this distinction can be sometimes artificial. Three types of localized granulomatous lesions can be distinguished: infectious granulomas, palisaded granulomas (granuloma annulare, necrobiosis lipoidica, and rheumatoid nodules), and foreign body granulomas. Disseminated granulomas can be divided into infectious, in particular tuberculosis, and noninfectious forms (autoimmune, neoplasia, etc.).

Keywords: granuloma, immune system, infection, inflammation, immunodeficiency

1. Introduction

Granulomatous diseases are not uncommon in daily clinical practice. Different etiologies (infection, autoimmunity, inflammation, foreign bodies, malignancy, metabolites, chemicals, etc.) can cause granulomatous lesions.

The differential diagnostic process for a granulomatous disease should always be made in light of interdisciplinary cooperation as it requires close collaboration between specialists including radiologists, internists, and pathologists.

Diagnostic procedures should be oriented to the clinical symptoms and should include blood analyses (liver and renal function control check, etc.), suggestive microbiological studies, and radiography (especially computed tomography or magnetic resonance imaging or positron emission tomography); the diagnosis of a granulomatous disease should always be confirmed by histopathology when possible, sampling for histology or cytology.

From a pathologic point of view, the lesions are divided into noninfectious and infectious granulomas. In the case of proven granulomatous inflammation, an infectious etiology (including mycobacteria, parasites, and fungi) should first be excluded.

From a clinical point of view, it is useful to separate granulomatosis into localized and disseminated forms, although this distinction can be sometimes artificial. Three types of localized granulomatous lesions can be distinguished: infectious granulomas, which are generally associated with localized infections, palisaded granulomas (granuloma annulare, necrobiosis lipoidica, and rheumatoid nodules), and foreign body granulomas. Disseminated granulomas can be divided into infectious (in particular tuberculosis) and noninfectious forms (autoimmune, neoplasia, etc.). These entities are discussed herein.

Granulomatous disorders are a heterogeneous group of diseases, the pathophysiological mechanism of which is still poorly understood. These are granulomatous inflammatory reactions to a wide variety of stimuli, including infections, systemic inflammations, neoplasia, metabolic disorders, and chemicals.

A granuloma is a specific form of inflammation involving mostly dendritic cells, T lymphocytes, and macrophages, which are the dominant cell type. Both innate and adaptive immunity are involved in this inflammatory process. From a clinical point of view, it is useful to separate granulomatosis into localized and disseminated forms, although this distinction may sometimes be artificial, because they often coexist. These are most frequently seen as pulmonary, hepatobiliary-splenic, gastrointestinal, renal, cerebral, and bone granulomas. From a pathogenic point of view, they are divided into noninfectious and infectious granulomas. Treatment is specific for each type.

2. Cutaneous localizad granulomatosis

The typical macroscopic skin lesion of cutaneous granulomatosis is characterized by an infiltrated painless rounded papule, which is well limited and reddish-pink and takes a yellowish color on diascopy, called apple jelly. Its surface is smooth or slightly squamous as there is generally no epidermal involvement [1].Three types of localized skin granulomatous lesions can be distinguished, namely, palisaded granulomas (like granuloma annulare, necrobiosis lipoidica, or rheumatoid nodules), infectious granulomas (which are generally associated with localized infections), and foreign body granulomas [1, 2].

2.1 Palisadic granulomas

This term corresponds to a histological description of a nodular inflammatory granulomatous lesion characterized by a central zone of altered connective tissue, surrounded by histiocytes dispersed in a palisaded form. The anomalies observed at the center of the granulomas generally make it possible to distinguish the different forms: mucin deposits in granuloma annulare, necrosis in necrobiosis lipoidica, and massive necrosis with fibrin deposits in rheumatoid nodules.

2.1.1 Granuloma annulare

This is the most commonly occurring form of cutaneous granulomas; two thirds of patients are under 30 years of age, with a male to female ratio of 2:1. Skin involvement predominates in the extremities and rarely involves the face. The localized form is the more common (75% of the cases) than disseminated disease. Disseminated granuloma annulare has also been described, sometimes isolated and sometimes reported to be in association with several conditions (i.e., paraneoplastic forms associated with solid organ tumors or lymphoma). In these patients, the skin picture is often atypical [1]. The dermatological expression is in the form of erythematous plaques, grouped in rings with centrifugal progression. These plaques are themselves made up of small, firm, and well-defined papules. These lesions are asymptomatic and generally located on the back of the hands and feet, wrists, ankles, and dorsolateral faces of the fingers. In the disseminated form, it is arranged symmetrically, mainly on the trunk and the extremities. The diagnosis is clinical, the cutaneous biopsy being useful in doubtful cases. Sometimes the biopsy itself leads to a regression of the lesion. The evolution of these skin lesions is unpredictable but generally benign. Typically, the skin lesions disappear spontaneously within a few months to 2–3 years. Treatment is usually indicated when the lesions are very generalized.

2.1.2 Necrobiosis lipoidica

Necrobiosis lipoidica is an idiopathic chronic granulomatosis, which usually occurs in young or middle-aged adults, with a male to female ratio of 1:3. It is associated with diabetes mellitus, although its development is not related to poor glycemic control.

Necrobiosis refers to a histological inflammation triggered by cell death, and lipoidica refers to the clinically yellowish appearance of the lesions due to lipid deposits secondary to collagen degeneration. The lesions present as bilateral painless papules or nodules, which widen progressively and converge into well-defined oval plaques with a raised erythematous border surrounding the central area, which is initially reddish and later becomes yellowish, smooth, and atrophic with telangiectasias and scarring. Over time, the plaque becomes indurated and adherent to the underlying osteoperiosteal planes, with a remaining active border. Isolated cases of squamous cell carcinomas have been reported in patients with large lesions.

2.1.3 Rheumatoid nodules

Rheumatoid nodules are the most frequent extra-articular manifestations of rheumatoid arthritis (RA). At least 20% of adult patients with RA have rheumatoid nodules. Patients with rheumatoid nodules are more often rheumatoid factor and anti-cyclic citrullinated peptide positive. Their presence in newly diagnosed patients can be considered as a clinical predictor of severe seropositive and erosive arthritis associated with extra-articular involvement, including rheumatoid vasculitis. They consist of deep dermo-hypodermic nodules of variable size (2 mm to 5 cm) adherent to the periosteum. Generally painless, these nodules can cause discomfort or pain when they ulcerate. The nodules tend to develop in outbreaks during the active phases of the disease and form subcutaneously, in the bursas and along the tendinous sheaths. Although they have been described in almost all regions and can occur in the viscera (lung, liver), these nodules are typically located at pressure points, such as on the extensor surface of the arm, the Achilles tendon, the ischial area, and on the flexor surfaces of the fingers. These lesions may develop gradually or abruptly and are usually associated with some symptoms of inflammation. A biopsy of the nodule may be necessary if the diagnosis is uncertain. Over time, rheumatoid nodules often disappear or regress, evolving sometimes, independent of treatment. Rheumatoid nodules appearing without clinical or biological rheumatic symptoms are most often deep granuloma annulare or pseudorheumatoid nodules, particularly in children and in the cephalic region [1, 2].

2.1.4 Lupus miliaris disseminatus faciei (acne agminata; necrotizing granulomatous rosacea)

Lupus miliaris disseminatus faciei is now believed to be a peculiar variant of rosacea. It presents with multiple reddish papules and nodules of the scalp and face, principally in young adults, and is centered on hair follicles, without pus formation. It usually persists for 2–3 years and then regresses, leaving residual scars [2].

2.2 Foreign body granulomas

Foreign body granulomas consist of an excessive cutaneous inflammatory response to any material in the dermis or subcutis (endogenous or exogenous). The clinical presentation and evolution depends on several factors: tissue response to the foreign body, anatomical site, penetration, composition, amount of material involved, quantity, and volume. They may appear as papules, nodules, or erythematous plaques which harden over time due to fibrosis. The time gap between entrance of the foreign body into the skin and appearance of granulomas is very variable, sometimes being as long as several years.

Among the endogenous substances, hair, calcifications, cholesterol crystals, or uric acid are common; while exogenous substances commonly include insects, silica (talc), beryllium, aluminum, or tattoo ink.

In recent years, the use of cosmetic materials and, in some cases, the implantation of medical material have been implicated in this regard. In recent years, a granulomatous and inflammatory systemic picture secondary to a foreign body reaction has been defined by diverse substances such as biomaterial injections and prostheses (mainly silicone, hyaluronic acid, acrylamides, and methacrylate compounds). The process is defined as autoimmune/inflammatory syndrome induced by adjuvants (ASIA) and is characterized by chronic fatigue, pyrexia, dry mouth, sleep disturbances, myalgia, myositis, muscle weakness, lymph nodes, arthralgia and/or arthritis, and foreign body-type granuloma, in the absence of any autoantibody, infection, or cancer. Symptoms may disappear after removal of the implant material [3].

2.3 Localized infectious granulomas

Infectious granulomas are usually chronic and localized skin infections, the agent being mycobacteria (tuberculosis or atypical mycobacteria), parasites (leishmaniasis), or fungi (cryptococcosis) in an immunocompromised host. With the exception of cutaneous leishmaniasis, granulomatous infections have to be considered as skin manifestations of systemic infections. They thus require systemic treatment directed toward the cause.

2.3.1 Cutaneous tuberculosis (TB)

Cutaneous tuberculosis (TB) accounts for less than 2% of all extrapulmonary tuberculosis manifestations and occurs in 10% of all patients with TB.

Skin manifestations of TB represent a clinical polymorphism that can be explained by various factors such as the pathogenicity of the bacterial strain, the immune status of the host, previous treatment, or local factors (i.e., proximity to lymph nodes). Localized forms include lupus vulgaris, a violaceous yellowish cutaneous plaque with serpiginous centrifugal extension, desquamation, and central atrophy, scrofuloderma (an erythemato-violaceous painless nodule, with suppuration as sign of per contiguitatem extension of ganglionic, osteoarticular), or epididymal tuberculosis or verrucous cutaneous tuberculosis (a keratotic plaque with irregular edges and dystrophic scarring on the skin of the hands). Cutaneous atypical mycobacteria infections have heterogeneous clinical appearance, including nodules, papules, plaques, pustules, abscess, and ulcers. *Mycobacterium marinum* is the most commonly involved strain. It causes skin and soft tissue infections after exposure to aquatic environments or marine animals ("tank granuloma"). Patients typically show clusters of nodules, ulcers, or verrucous plaques that may spread from the arms or legs in a sporotrichoid pattern. Mycobacterium chelonae is a rapidly growing mycobacterium that causes dark red nodules and, occasionally, abscesses. The infection is related to skin wounds due to penetration procedures (injection, liposuction, acupuncture, tattoos, etc.).

2.3.2 Cutaneous lesihmaniasis

Cutaneous leishmaniasis involves exposed body parts, causing nodules, ulcers, and scarring. Acute cutaneous leishmaniasis or East button is the most common form. The lesion, initially papular, rounded or oval, and asymptomatic or mildly pruritic, may be single or multiple and commonly located on the face or areas of uncovered skin. Gradually it takes a darker reddish tone while it infiltrates and increases in size. The surface is occasionally covered with furfuraceous scales and, in 1–3 months, is transformed into a nodular lesion or a deep infiltrated plaque. Chronic cutaneous leishmaniasis includes cases that exceed the duration of 1–2 years. The lesions are usually more polymorphic (large indurated plaques with papular borders, eczematiform, warty, keloidal, etc.), and the clinical difficulty of the diagnosis is due to the lower sensitivity of microscopic smear examination, the crops, and the histopathology.

2.4 Syndromic mucocutaneous granulomatous disorders

Cutaneous nonnecrotizing/necrobiotic granulomas may be part of syndromic complexes that include lesions in other organs and tissues as well. The two principal representatives of this group are the Melkersson-Rosenthal syndrome (orofacial mucocutaneous granulomatosis; cheilitis granulomatosa) and Blau syndrome [2].

The constituent signs of Melkersson-Rosenthal syndrome include the association of recurrent facial and/or lip edema, recurrent facial paralysis, and fissured tongue. It has been associated with Crohn's disease. Miescher's cheilitis granulomatous consists of the appearance of recurrent labial edema in one or both lips, which can be persistent. It has traditionally been considered as a monosymptomatic form of Melkersson-Rosenthal syndrome.

Blau syndrome is an autosomal-dominant autoinflammatory condition that includes granulomatous inflammation in the skin, together with granulomatous iridocyclitis and granulomatous arthritis with camptodactyly. It is related to mutations in the CARD15/NOD2 gene complex and may also have a linkage to Crohn's disease.

3. Systemic granulomatosis diseases

3.1 Infectious disseminated granuloma

Almost all infectious pathogens can induce granulomas (**Table 1**). Although the skin tends to be frequently affected, visceral involvement is usually coexisting, as is a systemic inflammatory process (fever, asthenia, etc.). There is no universal pattern of visceral or cutaneous involvement; the epidemiological and clinical context is essential, and physical history can provide data on the etiological agent.

Among infectious agents, mycobacteria are the most frequently involved. In tuberculosis and leprosy, there is either a true skin infection or tuberculids, which are regarded as a cutaneous hypersensitivity reaction to *Mycobacterium leprae* linked to the release of an antigen by an internal mycobacteria infectious focus. Skin tuberculid lesions are not contagious. The clinical manifestations of tuberculosis tuberculids are erythema nodosum, erythema induratum of Bazin, papulonecrotic tuberculids, lichen scrofulosorum, and lupus miliaris disseminatus faciei, whose differential diagnosis is granulomatous rosacea. Some agents have tropism due to specific viscera, such as bartonella due to the liver or the vascular affectation of syphilis. Some viruses are associated with specific vasculitic systemic processes, such as panarteritis nodosa in the case of hepatitis B or vasculitis cryoglobulinemia induced by the hepatitis C virus.

3.2 Noninfectious disseminated granuloma

There are many etiologies of noninfectious disseminated granulomas (**Table 2**). Possibly sarcoidosis is the prototype of these diseases, although it will not be

Bacteria	Virus	Fungi	Parasites
M. tuberculosis	Human immunodeficiency virus	*Candida* sp.	Toxoplasmosis
M. marinum	Epstein-Barr virus	*Aspergillus* sp.	*Leishmania* sp.
M. chelonae	Cytomegalovirus	Cryptococcosis	Bilharzia
M. avium (MAI)	Hepatitis B virus	Histoplasmosis	*Toxocara canis*
M. leprae	Hepatitis C virus	Blastomycosis	*Capillaria hepatica*
T. pallidum (syphilis)		Coccidioidomycosis	*Ascaris*
Salmonella sp.		Paracoccidioidomycosis	*Strongyloides*
Bartonella henselae		*Penicillium*	*Giardia lamblia*
Kleb. granulomatis (donovanosis)		*Sporothrix schenckii*	*Fasciola*
Listeriosis		*Pneumocystis jiroveci*	Schistosomiasis
Brucella			*Enterobius vermicularis* (pinworms)
Pasteurella			*Echinococcus granulosus*
Yersinia			*Echinococcus multilocularis*
Nocardia			
T. whipplei			
Rhodococcus equi			
Tularemia			
Melioidosis			
Coxiella burnetii			
Borrelia burgdorferi			

Table 1.
Common infectious diseases causing disseminated granulomatosis.

Immune-mediated inflammatory diseases

A. Organ specifies primarily

- Sarcoidosis
- Bronchogenic granulomatosis
- Inflammatory bowel disease
- Autoimmune hepatitis
- Primary biliary cirrhosis
- Primary sclerosing cholangitis
- Idiopathic eosinophilic gastroenteritis
- Chronic idiopathic inflammatory bowel disease

B. Systemic

- Lupus erythematosus
- Rheumatoid arthritis
- Polyarteritis nodosa
- Granulomatosis with polyangiitis (Wegener)
- Eosinophilic granulomatosis with polyangiitis (Churg-Strauss)

Neoplasia/clonal diseases

C. Hematological

- Lymphoma
  - Cutaneous: mycosis fungoides T-cell lymphoma (granulomatous)
  - Systemic:
  - Hodgkin
  - Non-Hodgkin
- Myelodysplastic syndrome

D. Solid tumors

- Primary: lung, breast, uterus, prostate, hepatocellular carcinoma
- Granulomatous reaction to metastases

Metabolic

E. Diabetes mellitus

F. Dyslipidemia

G. Thyroid disease

Toxic

H. Drugs: antihypertensives (angiotensin-converting enzyme inhibitors, calcium channel blockers, beta blockers, diuretics, hydralazine), hypolipidemic agents, anticonvulsants (phenytoin, topiramate), quinidine, antihistaminics, allopurinol, antimicrobials (nitrofurantoin, isoniazid), and others (beryllium, gold, copper toxicity, talc).

I. Immunotherapy and growth factors: interferon α, G-CSF, anti-TNF-α, IFN-α

Immunodeficiency

J. Common variable immunodeficiency

K. Wiskott-Aldrich syndrome

L. Chronic granulomatous diseases

Idiopathic

Table 2.
Causes of noninfectious systemic granulomas.

addressed in this chapter. Not all immune-mediated systemic processes should be assimilated as diseases capable of producing granulomas. For example, in the disease related to IgG4, although cases of pulmonary lymphomatoid granulomatosis associated with it have been described, two findings are extraordinary and practically discard it, namely, the presence of granulomas and the presence of a neutrophilic infiltrate [4, 5]. In this same sense we must refer to the diseases included in the so-called xanthogranulomatous diseases (Langerhans cell histiocytosis, Erdheim-Chester disease, Rosai-Dorfman disease, hemophagocytic lymphohistiocytosis, and juvenile xanthogranuloma) where space-occupying lesions can be seen in imaging techniques and a histiocytic infiltrate in biopsies, but rarely granulomas [6].

3.2.1 Chronic gastrointestinal and chronic biliary diseases

Granulomas have been reported in a small minority of patients with ulcerative colitis, Crohn's disease, and idiopathic eosinophilic gastroenteritis. It is unclear whether the granulomas associated with chronic idiopathic inflammatory bowel disease could be due to diseases such as primary sclerosing cholangitis or an adverse drug reaction. Granulomas may also be a feature of idiopathic eosinophilic enteritis involving the hepatobiliary tree by the disease.

Granulomas are reported very frequently (more than 50% in many series) in primary biliary cirrhosis cases. They may be portal or lobular, but are often associated with duct lesions. However, granulomas are also seen in a minority of cases in primary sclerosing cholangitis, in which they are usually well formed and non-necrotizing.

3.2.2 Vasculitis and collagen vascular diseases

Granulomas may involve the vasculature in collagen vascular diseases, like lupus erythematosus systemic, or more usually in vasculitic diseases including systemic necrotizing vasculitis and giant cell arteritis. Systemic necrotizing vasculitis is a group of heterogeneous diseases characterized clinically by a greater presentation and histologically by the presence of fibrinoid necrosis more intense than that seen in in other forms of vasculitis. Panarteritis nodosa is a vasculitis that characteristically affects the arteries of medium and small sizes. Vasculitis associated with antineutrophil cytoplasmic antibodies include granulomatosis accompanied by polyangiitis, microscopic polyarteritis, and granulomatous allergic angiitis.

3.2.3 Adverse drug reaction

After the skin, the liver is a frequent focus of granulomas secondary to drugs. Granulomas associated with adverse drug reactions may be well or poorly formed, but necrosis is very rare. Giant cells may be present, and there is a variable associated inflammatory infiltrate that may include lymphocytes, plasma cells, and eosinophils. There may be associated duct and/or vascular injury. The combination of granulomatous inflammation with significant hepatocellular injury strongly suggests drug-associated liver injury [7].

3.2.4 Primary immunodeficiency

As in severely immunosuppressed patients (transplant patients, advanced HIV, etc.), cases of primary immunodeficiencies and systemic granulomatous complications, either primary or following opportunistic infections, may appear.

Common variable immunodeficiency comprises a heterogeneous group of diseases characterized by a significant hypogammaglobulinemia of unknown cause, failure to produce specific antibodies after immunization, and susceptibility to bacterial infections, but others develop complications, like granulomas or autoimmune diseases. Sarcoid-like granulomas are also well described in the liver, spleen, and lung in patients with common variable immunodeficiency [8]. This involvement is usually associated with other autoimmune manifestations and has a worse prognosis.

Chronic granulomatous disease is a rare primary immunodeficiency caused by an inherited defect in the genes encoding any of the NADPH oxidase components responsible for the respiratory burst of phagocytic leukocytes. The NADPH oxidase is responsible for the production of reactive oxygen species (ROS) in the activated phagocyte ("respiratory burst"). When present, mutations on the NAPDH oxidase genes do not allow ROS production, making the neutrophils of these patients incapable of destroying pathogens. These patients are especially susceptible to infections by staphylococcus, fungi and some gram-negative bacteria. The main clinical manifestations include recurrent life-threatening episodes of lymphadenitis, abscess, pneumonias, osteomyelitis, granuloma formation, and sepsis [8].

3.2.5 Interstitial granulomatous dermatitis

It is important to recognize interstitial granulomatous dermatitis, because although it can sometimes occur as an isolated skin disease, it is often associated with a systemic disease, which marks the prognosis of the patient; thus an active study should be carried out [4]. Ackerman first described this rare type of dermatitis in 1993. Although the original manifestation has been described as subcutaneous linear nodules (also known as rope sign), later reports showed a quite heterogeneous clinical spectrum ranging from hyperpigmented, erythematous papules, subcutaneous plaques, and annular lesions to firm red purplish nodules. The lesions are usually asymptomatic, but can be slightly pruritic or painful. The histopathological examination confirms the diagnosis and is characterized by a dense and diffuse interstitial infiltrate in the reticular dermis, composed of histiocytes in a palisade arrangement, sometimes with necrobiosis of collagen and neutrophils and eosinophils. Interstitial granulomatous dermatitis has been associated with various systemic diseases, including autoimmune diseases such as rheumatoid arthritis (the most common), systemic sclerosis, or lupus erythematosus. Recently, a case has been reported in association with primary biliary cholangitis. However, other etiologies have been described in isolated cases including malignancy or drugs (angiotensin-converting enzyme inhibitors, calcium channel blockers, beta blockers, diuretics, TNF-α blockers, etc.) [1, 4].

4. Diagnostic approach

The diagnostic approach must be structured, and the analytical, microbiological, or radiological tests must be adapted to the epidemiological factors of the patient's clinical history, as well as to the results of the physical examination. Obtaining a biopsy, both for histological and microbiological studies, is fundamental. In cases of uncertain etiology, close monitoring should be carried out, given the association of granulomas with potentially serious diseases (**Table 3**).

Medical history

- Comorbidities (autoimmune disease, diabetes, immunosuppression)
- Drugs or foreign body or water exposure
- Travels
- Risk exposures (sexual, parenteral drugs, etc.)

Physical examination: Clinical sign-associated diseases

Biopsy (depending on the affected organ and accessibility)

- Histology
- Microbiology
    - Culture (bacteria, mycobacteria)
    - PCR (mycobacteria, parasites, etc.)

Laboratory testing

- Complete blood count, ESR, CRP, creatinine, calcemia, liver enzymes, LDH, glycemia, cholesterol, triglycerides, TSH/T4, serum protein electrophoresis, ANA, rheumatoid factor, angiotensin-converting enzyme
- Serology for HIV, syphilis, hepatitis B and C, and others according to clinical suspicion

Mantoux or interferon gamma release assays for TB

Radiological tests

- Chest X-ray and abdomen and pelvic ultrasound
- Others according to clinical suspicion: CT scan, PET-CT, etc.

Table 3.
Diagnostic approach to granulomatous diseases.

5. Conclusion

- Granulomatous disorders are a heterogeneous group of diseases, including infections, systemic inflammations, neoplasia, metabolic disorders, and chemicals.
- An adequate clinical approach, together with physical examination and basic analysis, can guide the diagnostic process. However, biopsy of the lesion is usually fundamental.
- The histological type of granuloma is important in the etiological diagnosis, to optimize both treatment and follow-up.

Conflict of interest

No conflict of interests declared.

Author details

Angel Robles-Marhuenda
Unidad de Enfermedades Autoinmunes Sistémicas, Servicio de Medicina Interna, Hospital Universitario La Paz, Madrid, Spain

*Address all correspondence to: aroblesmarhuenda@gmail.com

References

[1] Terziroli B, Mainetti C, Peeters MA, Laffitte E. Cutaneous granulomatosis: A comprehensive review. Clinical Reviews in Allergy and Immunology. 2018;**54**:131-146. DOI: 10.1007/s12016-017-8666-8

[2] Wick MR. Granulomatous & histiocytic dermatitides. Seminars in Diagnostic Pathology. 2017;**34**:301-311. DOI: 10.1053/j.semdp.2016.12.003

[3] Alijotas-Reig J, Esteve-Valverde E, Gil-Aliberas N, Garcia-Gimenez V. Autoimmune/inflammatory syndrome induced by adjuvants—ASIA—related to biomaterials: Analysis of 45 cases and comprehensive review of the literature. Immunologic Research. 2017;**66**:120-140. DOI: 10.1007/s12026-017-8980-5

[4] Deshpande V, Zen Y, Chan JK, Yi EE, Sato Y, Yoshino T, et al. Consensus statement on the pathology of IgG4-related disease. Modern Pathology. 2012;**25**:1181-1192. DOI: 10.1038/modpathol.2012.72

[5] Lamps LW. Hepatic granulomas: A review with emphasis on infectious causes. Archives of Pathology & Laboratory Medicine. 2015;**139**:867-875. DOI: 10.5858/arpa.2014-0123-RA

[6] Bourm KS, Menias CO, Ali K, Alhalabi K, Elsayes KM. Spectrum of xanthogranulomatous processes in the abdomen and pelvis: A pictorial review of infectious, inflammatory, and proliferative responses. AJR. American Journal of Roentgenology. 2017;**208**:475-484. DOI: 10.2214/AJR.16.17075

[7] Dodiuk-Gad RP, Shear NH. Granulomatous drug eruptions. Dermatologic Clinics. 2015;**33**:525-539. DOI: 10.1016/j.det.2015.03.015

[8] Picard C, Al-Herz W, Bousfiha A, Casanova J-L, Chatila T, Conley ME, et al. Primary immunodeficiency diseases: An update on the classification from the International Union of Immunological Societies Expert Committee for Primary Immunodeficiency 2015. Journal of Clinical Immunology. 2015;**35**:696-726. DOI: 10.1007/s10875-015-0201-1